To
Grady Turner
Best Wishes for
Good health &
a long happy
useful life

Sincerely
Joe Michaels MD
6-21-89

JOE D. NICHOLS, M.D.
President, Natural Food Associates
and
James Presley

"PLEASE, DOCTOR, *DO* SOMETHING!"

A Modern Physician Looks at Health and Nutrition

THE DEVIN-ADAIR COMPANY
Old Greenwich, Connecticut

1st Printing, April 1972
2nd Printing, January 1973
3rd Printing, July 1973
4th Printing, October 1975
5th Printing, December 1976

Introduction

This autobiography of Dr. Joe Nichols will help many individuals to attain and maintain optimal health.

It comes at a most opportune time.

It is the common wish of all mankind to have optimal health. Most, however, do not realize that the physician is only a repairman. The individual, either willfully or through ignorance, violates the rules of hygiene. He then takes the resulting diseased body to the doctor to be made whole again. This can never be done, but the physician does, in these times, perform a remarkable repair job so that the impaired body can run a while longer. Each individual citizen must be responsible for attaining and maintaining the health of his own body. No one can do this for him.

> "Virtue" says Carrel, "is to avoid sin against Nature; it is to keep healthy and manly; to respect life in one's self and in others; to try to propagate it in the best possible conditions; to protect the integrity of one's physical being against undermining or intoxicants; and that of one's moral being against falsehood, futility and calumny."

This demands what Dr. Nichols calls a "Concept of Totality." So we find the author active in soil, water and forest conservation, associating himself with Friends of the Land, Biodynamic Farming and Gardening Association, and Natural Food Associates. Someone has put all this very succinctly when he wrote, "In the consideration of Man in relation to everything about him—his attempts to organize his environment to his benefit as well as his attempt to adapt himself more effectively to it; also the impact of each factor in the environment upon him, we assemble into a new discipline meteorology, climatology, geology, agronomy, agriculture in all of its aspects, medicine and its basic sciences, the social sciences and business administration. In fact, Ecology of Man becomes an attempt to focus all that Man has learned in the past centuries upon the present problems of human adaptation to his own personal environment."

Here, then, in this volume a physician relates his experiences in an attempt to adapt himself to the busy life of a Texas physician and surgeon and to correct, as far as it is humanly possible, his own impaired body so that he could and has led a very active professional life and, at the same time, be one of the founders of Natural Food Associates and become its leader. In this way, Dr. Nichols has been able to convey the message of real "Health Care" to thousands throughout the United States, Canada and Mexico.

We, in Natural Food Associates, know that the author's message is valid and, if put to use, will bring health to all who read it.

JONATHAN FORMAN, A.B., M.D., F.A.C.A.

Preface

America, land of the free? It is a myth!

Most babies born in America today do not have the freedom to breathe poison-free air.

Most babies born in America today do not have the freedom to drink poison-free water.

Most babies born in America today do not have the freedom to eat poison-free food.

Most babies born in America today do not even have the freedom to nurse the mother's breast without being poisoned with DDT.

One of seven babies born in America today comes into the world with a birth defect.

As a result of the loss of these freedoms, most babies born in America today do not have the freedom to be healthy.

America, land of the free? It is a myth.

We must regain these lost freedoms and this book is an attempt to outline a way of life that will do just that.

America is one of the sickest and worst-fed nations on earth. All types of metabolic diseases are increasing at an alarming rate. Billions of dollars have been spent in an attempt to control cancer, heart disease, diabetes, arthritis, and other metabolic diseases; yet all these diseases continue to increase, and almost nothing is being done to prevent them. The greatest single cause of metabolic disease is malnutrition and the poisons in our food. We have an abundance of food in America, but it is of very low quality. The vital minerals and vitamins have been removed from too much of our food. We are facing a metabolic, as well as ecological, crisis. Recognizing that "the whiter the bread, the quicker you are dead" is a pithy, accurate warning, I maintain that one of America's greatest needs today is a good loaf of bread.

Proper nutrition will prevent most of our metabolic diseases. And what is proper nutrition? Proper nutrition can be found only in natural, poison-free food grown on fertile soil, eaten fresh, and not overcooked.

What is natural food? What is fertile soil? This book answers these questions and will tell you how to get proper nutrition for you and your family.

I have a personal stake in promoting good nutrition. I have two sons, Joe Dan Nichols, Jr., and David Nichols.

Dan is a physician and has joined my clinic here in Atlanta. David is a dentist. Both of them understand the importance of the concept of total nutrition. They graduated from the University of Tennessee Medical and Dental Schools in Memphis.

I will never forget the night when Dan called and announced the great news that we were going to be grandparents. I usually go to bed about 10 p.m. and sleep until 6:30 a.m. But on that night about 3 a.m. I heard a voice that brought me to my feet. I heard, as clearly as I have ever heard anything, a voice say, "Grandpa, please get up and do something." I heard my unborn grandchild say, "Please, Dr. Joe, I don't want to be born prematurely and never see outside a hospital. Please, Doctor, I don't want to be born with a birth defect. Please, Grandpa, get up and do something." I heard my unborn grandchild say, "Please, Dr. Joe, I don't want to be born with cancer. Please, Doctor, *do* something!"

The cry of my unborn grandchild motivated this book. This book is dedicated to him and to thousands of others like him.

JOE D. NICHOLS, M.D.

Atlanta, Texas
January 30, 1972

Contents

I.

A Personal Genesis

We are a nation of sick people.

I almost died, the day I learned this. I learned it the hard way, by becoming one of those people. But, paradoxically, the experience saved my life, for out of the agony and travail of that personal crisis and subsequent intellectual odyssey, I learned why we are a nation of sick people, and what we can do about it. What I learned may save your life too, and the lives of your children.

On May 23, 1946, I experienced what millions of other Americans, and thousands of my fellow doctors, have gone through. I got sick. I got so sick I thought I was going to die.

I was as busy, back in 1946, as I had ever been and this, later, was cited as the reason I became sick. Very early in life, as a boy in Parkdale, Arkansas, I had become accustomed to working hard and for long hours. I had not let up after getting out of the University of Arkansas Medical School. Since 1933 I had been practicing medicine in Atlanta, Texas, (population now: 5,534) and was an owner of a twelve-bed hospital, where I also was the surgeon. I kept further busy in business and civic matters. I was chairman of the board of the Atlanta National Bank and president of the Atlanta Chamber of Commerce. It kept me going from early in the morning until late at night.

As if there were not enough to keep me busy, I had just

bought a 1,000-acre farm. Just improving and managing that farm alone would have been enough to keep me occupied most of my waking hours. The land was so poor it would hardly grow weeds; I had paid $10 an acre for it, and it was not worth that much. But as enthusiastically as I had gone into anything else, I was determined to make that farm a showplace. Admittedly, I had my work cut out for me. I borrowed $20,000 and bought a fine herd of registered Shorthorn cattle. I was going to be a real "do-gooder" and put some good bulls in the country. The cows had become fat and healthy from a fertile Red River farm in East Texas. But at my farm they began to lose weight immediately. They got sick, and most of them died. I poured additional thousands of dollars into them, buying feed and medicine and paying for the frequent services of a veterinarian. They kept dying. As a physician and banker, I had no complaints about success and my status in life, but as an apprentice cattleman, I had a long way to go.

The day I got sick I was attending a regional chamber of commerce meeting in an East Texas city about 100 miles away. The secretary of our local chamber went with me. We had to leave home early that morning, so both he and I skipped breakfast. But we both felt fine when we took off, and we bought a new box of big black cigars and set out exuberantly to enjoy ourselves.

We held the meeting in a Methodist Church, most memorable to me today for its hard benches where we sat all morning while listening to the reports and speeches. By noon we were starved, and we welcomed the heavy lunch of ham, barbecue meat, beans, white bread, and pie. This was what I considered an excellent meal. In those days I ate white bread, refined salt, shortening, white sugar, and dry cereals like everybody else did. They were all ingredients of a balanced meal, weren't they? Like most of my colleagues that day, I ate ravenously. We agreed it was a great lunch.

After eating, we were all taken to see a new brick plant in the city. I was particularly interested in the manufacturing process, because we had a similar industry back home. Consequently I strayed off by myself to take a closer look at the brick ovens, while the other men strolled off in another direction.

It was extremely hot by the ovens, which was possibly one reason the tour had not been routed in as closely as I went. The heat of the ovens, added to that of the burning late May afternoon Texas sun, made it very hot there, indeed.

As I was studying the ovens, with the heat gushing out from them, suddenly a great pain struck me in the chest. It was the most terrific pain I had ever felt in my life.

I fell to the floor, afraid to move. Paralyzed by fear, incapacitated by pain, I was afraid the pain would get worse—which seemed impossible—and brusquely snuff out my life. Before that day I had had some chest pains, but, as many laymen and even doctors are also guilty of doing, I had refused to believe it might be heart trouble. Now I had no doubts at all. I *knew* I had had a heart attack. I was just lying there, waiting, hoping it would subside, trusting everything would come out all right.

My friend who had come with me, missing me, turned and saw me lying on the ground, a couple of hundred yards behind them. He and another man ran over to where I was. By now the pain was letting up a little.

"What's the matter? What happened? he asked frantically. He had no idea what was wrong. Had I burned myself on the ovens? Had I somehow broken a leg?

"I have a severe chest pain," I managed to say.

"We've got to get you to a doctor!" he said.

"No, I'll be all right," I said, a statement no sensible layman should make, much less a doctor. The truth was, I was afraid to move. This fear is common to heart patients: they are afraid the pain will get worse if they move.

I lay still for about ten minutes, until the pain had subsided. My friend insisted that he take me to a doctor. I declined, for the same reason a layman might have: I didn't know a physician there and I didn't want to go to a strange doctor. But I didn't tell my friend that. So he put me into the car, and he drove me home.

I knew I was sick, and I knew I was seriously ill. I was a doctor. I had seen enough patients to recognize the symptoms. Furthermore, I had a pretty good idea of the odds on a heart case like mine. They weren't good. I was in the same predicament of many patients I had treated, and it was not comforting to know that many another man had experienced exactly what I had gone through that day, for many of them had died. There was no reason to think I had a golden ticket to survival. Frankly, I was scared.

For several days I did nothing. Nothing at all. I lay around the house, resting, trying to relax. I let my practice go, as well as all my other responsibilities. The pain I had felt as I lay on the ground that afternoon had been burned indelibly into my psyche. I knew how close death had come, how close it could come again.

I went to a cardiologist in Dallas. He took an EKG, or electrocardiograph reading of my heart tracings. Beneath my customary joviality I awaited the results as anxiously as any of his other patients.

In a sense, he reported good news. He could find no evidence that I had suffered a coronary.

But he also said, "You're a doctor. You know what's going on. Slow down. Take a month off and rest."

He suggested a salt-free diet, which was the limit of his dietary instructions, and he prescribed nitroglycerin tablets. Nitroglycerin dilates the blood vessels, which makes circulation easier, with less strain on the heart. But nitroglycerin also dilates the vessels in the head. In some patients this causes headaches. This is what it did to me. I would get terrific headaches when I took the tablets. And because the headaches became more and more painful, I would postpone taking the tablets until it seemed absolutely necessary to prevent heart pain.

I was thirty-seven years old.

My heart disease and my 1,000-acre East Texas farm are both inextricably intertwined in my life. The resurrection of my poor, worn-out soil is intimately related to my own escape from coronary disaster. And even as I lay about home, doing nothing, I thought about the farm.

By then, June had come. Summer was upon us, and my wife and I decided to take a trip away from it all. Our two small sons, Dan and David, were out of school for the summer. Mildred's sister was married to General Archie Olds of the Air Force and so we drove to California to visit the Olds for three weeks.

It was while we were driving to California, crossing the Arizona desert, that we finally came up with a name for the 1,000-acre farm. One day Mildred suddenly snapped her fingers and exclaimed:

"I've got it!"

"You've got what?"

"The name! The name for our farm. Jonica Farm. Jo-nic-a. Jo-nic for Joe Nichols. A for Allday. Jonica." Allday was Mildred's maiden name.

The name stuck.

In California I lay around and rested, and hoped I would recover. I had plenty of time to think, as we visited General and Mrs. Olds, and I had time to think when we returned to Texas later in the month. And I had plenty to think about. Why was I having heart disease at thirty-seven? I had thought it was a disorder for old men. Now I knew better and my eyes had been opened, and questions grew in my mind. I knew the orthodox way of dealing with heart disease, and it didn't leave me bubbling with optimism. I had been a physician long enough, and had seen enough patients, to know the end of the road wasn't far ahead. My prognosis was not good. There had to be another answer, something that hadn't been taught me in medical school. What was it? Where could I find the answers to the questions I had never asked before?

Most people, including myself, blamed my illness on my working too hard under too much stress. Others blamed it on the big noon meal and the heat from the brick ovens. But it was hard to accept so simply that these factors alone had brought me to the brink of eternity at thirty-seven. Yet it was the best I knew. I went back to work after taking a month off. I kept taking the nitroglycerin and I kept getting terrible headaches that were almost as bad as the chest pains the tablets prevented. It left me with the utmost respect and consideration for the patient with a coronary; a little coronary is bad enough.

About this time somehow I got on the free list of what is now *Organic Gardening and Farming,* a magazine published by the late J. I. Rodale in Emmaus, Pennsylvania. I had no idea how I got on the free list, but I had a 1,000-acre farm, poor as it was, and so I didn't throw the magazine away. I read some of the articles and the ads. Organic farming. Diet of organically-grown food. Quackery, I thought. I had been taught about diet. I was a doctor and had advised hundreds of patients on diets. One statement in the magazine proclaimed: "People who eat natural food grown on fertile soil don't have heart disease." Quackery of the worst sort, I thought; after all, the editor of the magazine was not a doctor. What else was this but pure quackery and food faddism?

I had accepted the subscription with many negative thoughts. If I had not been desperately ill, I probably would never have even read the magazine. But the heart trouble had wedged open my mind, just a crack. Natural food grown on fertile soil? Well, it was food quackery, all right, but something—no doubt the memory of my heart pain as I lay on the ground by the brick ovens—made me read. And the quotation, "People who eat natural food grown on fertile soil don't have heart disease," stuck in my mind, quackery or not.

But two questions nagged at me. What is natural food? What is fertile soil?

I had an A.B. degree, an M.D. degree, was fairly intelligent, had read a lot, now owned a farm, but I didn't know what natural food was. Like many another American who hadn't really investigated the subject, I thought "natural food" meant wheat germ and blackstrap molasses and that all natural food addicts were food faddists, quacks, and nuts. I thought you made land fertile by dumping commercial fertilizer on it.

There were three books advertised in the magazine that caught my eye. The main reason I became interested in the books was that I was sick and I was willing to consider anything at all that would help me get well. So I ordered them. Another reason I thought I might want to read them was to help with the big farm that seemed to be getting worse off. I was losing money on it. Although I didn't think of it that way at the time, the farm was sicker than I was, or at least as sick.

One was a book by Sir Albert Howard called *An Agricultural Testament*. Another was *Nutrition and the Soil* by Sir Lionel Picton, and the third one, *Nutrition and Natural Health,* was by Sir Robert McCarrison, a very famous nutritionist whose work in India I had heard of. All three men were British scientists. They had been knighted by the British crown. They were respected.

I read those three books, and I've never been the same since. Sir Albert Howard was an authority on the subjects of both agriculture and nutrition. Each of the other two men was recognized in his field. I had to admit that these men were not quacks or food faddists. They not only knew what they were talking about, they were acknowledged as experts by others who should know. This realization opened up a whole new vista in my life. For the first time since I had had my heart symptoms I could see hope dawning. I became very excited.

Although these three books didn't answer all of my questions, they gave me a good idea of what I wanted to know and they gave me strong indications of my two questions, What is natural food, and What is fertile soil? Roughly, using just plain common sense, natural food means food that still has in it the natural vitamins and minerals and enzymes that an all-wise Creator put there. Nothing taken out, nothing put in. A fertile soil is a soil in which the conditions are optimum for the growth of soil micro-organisms. The Ph, or alkaline-acid balance, must be right. A fertile soil is a *living* soil. The soil micro-organism is the chef that feeds the plants. It is the doctor that produces the antibiotic that makes a healthy plant.

In other words, all of the ideas I had held for so long were wrong. Commercial fertilizers didn't make land fertile; over the years it killed the land. Natural food wasn't just wheat germ and blackstrap molasses; it was all the foods we needed, grown without commercial fertilizers or poisons.

Proper nutrition, I learned, means *natural, poison-free food grown on fertile soil, eaten fresh and not overcooked.* I wish I could have learned that very simple fact while I was in medical school. Instead, I had gone until 1946 eating junk food just like everyone else. I ate refined salt, hydrogenated fats, white flour, white sugar, and the commercial dry cereals, not knowing that such so-called foods were leading me directly into heart disease.

Those three writers had convinced me that the big answer to metabolic disease, whether it was heart trouble or cancer or diabetes, was natural, poison-free food grown on fertile soil. Out of the conviction I logically developed after reading and thinking about those three books, it became clear to me that I had developed heart disease as a result of poor nutrition. I had a lifetime of eating junk foods behind me. This was the chief culprit, although stress, overwork, and overeating had certainly played their parts. But I knew that, fortunately, the heart has a tremendous capacity to regenerate itself, if a person learns to avoid junk foods and returns to proper nutrition. This I set out to do.

I was determined to find the answers, in depth, to my questions, What is natural food and what is fertile soil? At the time I had been a member of the Texas Medical Association's House of Delegates for many years. The TMA Library was in Fort Worth. The librarian was a good friend of mine. One day I drove over to Fort Worth, getting up in the middle of the night to drive the 200 miles from Atlanta. I thought the TMA Library would have the answers to my questions, somewhere in those honeycombs of published technical medical knowledge.

I was at the library at eight a.m. when it opened.

"I came to find the answers to two questions," I said. "One, what is natural food? Two, what is fertile soil?"

The librarian was very helpful. There was a large reading room with a long table. She and another lady kept bringing me books on nutrition as fast as I could go through them. I looked through the medical literature all day, but I couldn't find the answers to my questions. On the contrary, most of the material they brought me was what I had been taught before—the modern, orthodox teachings—and it was in disagreement with what I had learned in those three books.

I knew then I would have to look elsewhere. Eagerly I examined every opportunity to further enlighten myself. I had a feeling it was going to save my life.

II.

A New Road to Health

I have said it many times, and it is true: the best thing that ever happened to me was heart disease. If it hadn't been for that, I would have been dead long ago. But because of it I began seeking answers I had never bothered about before.

During this time, somebody sent me a copy of the program of the annual convention of the American Academy of Applied Nutrition, which was to be held in Pasadena, California. The caliber of men on the program impressed me. They had physicians, dentists, and men with Ph.D. degrees as leaders of the organization, all men with training and experience. I was still at the beginning of my quest for the right preventive answers, and I was willing to travel anywhere and read anything and listen to anyone, as long as I thought there was a chance to find, or even to stumble upon, the truth. And I was desperate in my search to find some way to stop the frightening chest pains I still suffered. A big coronary was headed in my direction and I knew it. I decided to go to California.

In Pasadena I met some of the top scientists and nutritionists in the world. There were men and women who knew the answers to the questions I had been asking. They were physicians, dentists, and scientists with all the various doctoral degrees: M.D., D.D.S., Ph.D. I listened to them and I began to find answers. I met Dr. William Albrecht from the University of Missouri, an agricultural authority. Dr. Royal Lee, without a doubt, knew more about nutrition than any other man I've ever met. Men like Dr. Jonathan Forman, an allergist from Columbus, Ohio, had known about proper nutrition for years and years.

I also met there some of the biggest food faddists and quacks in the world. Some were pushing "miracle" foods. Others were selling political and religious ideas. There were people who could tell you how to go to heaven, how to go to hell, or anywhere in between. I met a metaphysicist that I felt was, to put it as plainly as I can, nuts. In a few short days I was exposed to both sides of the food issue, as I have been ever since. On one side was *bona fide*, scientifically-sound nutrition; on the other, *bona fide* faddism. I came away from there with an education, for sure.

When I returned home from Pasadena I was on my way. I became an organic farmer, and I started eating natural foods. I was convinced that natural food was the way, but I hadn't reached the point where I had eradicated from my diet some of the worst of our twentieth-century processed foods. For instance, I still ate crackers and a few other junk foods. It takes time to overcome decades of personal habit, and eating is as personalized as anything we do. I was still learning, and I was still in the process of recognizing and discarding junk foods.

Natural foods became a passion with me. I had seen the light, and I was understandably eager to tell others. I started ordering natural food from as far off as Pennsylvania, California, and Florida, wherever I could find organically-grown, poison-free food. My chest pains vanished. I threw away my nitroglycerin tablets and my headaches with them. I felt better than I ever had before. I had found the secret of good health, if not of life itself, and it had saved my life. I started making speeches to any group that would listen. I was anxious to share my good fortune. Furthermore, I was determined to make Jonica Farm a successful, shining example of natural farming.

People laughed. They made fun of the doctor who had gone to extremes and whose farm would surely break him financially. But nothing deterred me. What I lacked in precise knowledge I made up for with enthusiasm and exuberance. In the vernacular of my East Texas homeland, I was a "real, sure-nuff goin' joker." I was ready to save the world. I knew a good thing, and I wasn't keeping any secrets. I wanted the world to know. How else could I save it?

I bought a red truck and had this legend painted on the doors in yellow:

Jonica Farm
Organic Vegetables

When the red truck with "Jonica Farm" emblazoned on its sides drove into Atlanta, all the farmers laughed. The good doctor was learning his lesson the hard way, and they enjoyed it.

I made mistakes, but I learned from them. I was determined to grow my own food and never again to eat overprocessed, poisoned, degerminated junk foods. I became so enthusiastic about it all that I had to tell every patient I saw this whole story of natural food grown on fertile soil. It is very time-consuming, telling the whole story and translating this into specific recommendations for the daily diet, and many of them did not want to listen. I warned them of white bread, especially. I tried to educate them on the virtues of the wholewheat bread, organically grown—a brown diet. Soon they had given me a nickname. They called me "Dr. Brown." As I heard the story, patients said, very often, "There's no reason going to Dr. Nichols. He won't give you any medicine. He'll just try to put you on that 'brown diet.'" Some even said I was making money out of it. That wasn't true. I was losing money. I lost most of my practice—which it took me years to recover.

What happened to me, a smalltown doctor in Texas, could have happened to anyone else anywhere else in this country. Heart disease recognizes no geographic limits, no professional exemptions, no age or sex barriers. Just as easily, my case could have been that of a salesman in California or a newspaperman in New York or an automobile factory technician or executive in Michigan or a farmer in Florida. More so than they, I had thought I knew all the answers about diet and good health. I was a physician. I was supposed to know. But my heart trouble had proved me wrong, and that had given me an extra shock. The threat of losing your life, the idea of losing all you have worked for, including your wife, children and friends, is bad enough. It is a further shock, a double shock, to discover that which you have believed all your life is in error. Yet it took the double shock to save my life, by sending me on a relentless search for the truth.

What I did to salvage my life and health can, also, be done by anyone else anywhere else. Although I was fortunate enough to own a large farm and had the means to grow my own food, it is also possible to have natural, poison-free food that is grown on fertile soil, wherever you live, whoever you are. Even if you live in an apartment complex in the biggest city in the world, you may be out of touch with nature, but you don't have to be out of touch with health.

I intend to tell you how to get natural, poison-free food grown on fertile soil, no matter how old you are, which sex you are, what color you are, no matter where you live—north, south, east, or west, on an isolated farm or in a big city apartment. This book, I hope to make obvious, is for *everybody*. I still think there's time to save the world.

America today—I think you will agree with me when you have reflected on the evidence to be presented in this book—is suffering from a biological blight. We are facing metabolic disaster in this country. We call ourselves the best-nourished, healthiest nation on the face of the globe. Nothing could be farther from the truth. We are a nation of sick people. Whether we officially acknowledge it or not, the state of our people's health is a national disgrace and we are in crisis, at this very moment. And, moreover, what is true here is being duplicated in many other nations all over the world, for the American way of nutrition, sadly, is becoming the way of millions of foreigners.

Reflect on these facts for a moment. Heart disease is rampaging through America. It is our Public Enemy Number One. It is the leading cause of death among Americans. Fifty years ago, coronary thrombosis was rarely seen by a physician. Today it strikes even in the young. It used to be routine procedure for newspaper obituary writers to doublecheck on causes of death among men forty or younger; there was a chance of overlooking a violent death that might make a news story. Today, such checking is usually a waste of time; chances are, the young man died of heart disease. A report on 1,600 autopsies showed that in every one of the patients past the age of *three years*, there was already disease in the aorta, the main artery of the body that carries blood from the left ventricle of the heart to all organs and parts except the lungs. In every patient past the age of *twenty*, disease was already in the coronary artery. This should be evidence enough that practically everybody in the United States today has cardiovascular disease. I think maybe everybody's got it. We have an epidemic. Not only is heart disease the leading cause of death in this country, but it is increasing each year, despite the millions and millions of dollars the government contributes for research, despite the millions the American people pour out to the American Heart Association. All this money hasn't changed the basic fact or the status of heart disease as a killer.

Now, let's take cancer. When I graduated from the University of Arkansas Medical School in 1932, cancer was almost unknown in children. It was a medical rarity. This is a brief span in man's life, from 1932 to the present. It is nothing in the millions of years man has been here. Yet today we have an epidemic of cancer. Cancer—and this is an astounding statistic—is now the leading cause of death, after accidents, in children under fifteen years of age! Babies are being *born* with cancer. It no longer is a rarity for a young person to die of cancer. According to the American Cancer Society, *cancer will eventually strike one of every four Americans now living.* One out of four! This is an unheard-of ratio, and a dramatic, new development.

On top of this, the National Foundation (March of Dimes)—and I don't think anyone would dispute their figures—tells us that *one out of seven* children will be born with birth defects.

And recently we have learned that one out of 350 babies will die a crib death—that baffling case when a baby goes to sleep at night apparently healthy and, inexplicably, is found dead in his crib the next morning.

Diabetes was almost unknown in children when I graduated from medical school. We used the Benedict test then, in which glucose in urine reduces blue alkaline copper sulfate to red cuprous oxide. There is not a more accurate test today. Today diabetes is common in children, and it is increasing by leaps and bounds.

Today one out of every sixteen children is born mentally retarded, and we know why. Malnutrition and the poisons in our foods are not the only causes, but they are the chief causes.

Although millions of dollars are being spent to add poison sodium fluoride to the public water supply, dental caries are raging. Yet we could prevent caries easily. We already know how. My dentist son wrote a paper in which he summed it up in one sentence: "To prevent dental caries, all you have to do is *keep your mouth clean and eat right.*"

Gallstones, kidney stones, arthritis, multiple sclerosis, muscular dystrophy—all of these plague Americans in increasing numbers. The list could go on and on.

Is this the roll call of a healthy nation?

Can a nation call itself healthy when one of four must expect to get cancer, when three out of four who get cancer will die of it?

Is early detection the only hope for that one out of four who gets cancer?

If that's the best we can look forward to, then God save us! It's a bleak road ahead for the coming generations, and for their children, who likely will be born with several metabolic strikes against them.

I am very proud of my profession. I have a son in my clinic and I hope my grandson will someday follow in our footsteps. I have another son who is a dentist. The medical profession can point with pride at progress that has been made in many fields. We can now save lives that would have been lost in the days when I was in medical school. Great advances have been made in surgical technique, in anesthesiology, and in the prevention of certain infectious diseases. We rarely see tetanus, for instance. I have not seen a case of tetanus since I got out of medical school. Men and women who formerly would have died with pneumonia are alive today as a result of our antibiotics.

Pneumonia used to be the Public Enemy Number One in America. It killed more persons than did anything else. Today it is far down the list. Heart disease now is Public Enemy Number One. This, and the fact that heart disease is on the increase, demonstrates that we have made little progress in the solution of our metabolic diseases. Gallstones, kidney stones, arthritis, diabetes, cancer, multiple sclerosis, muscular dystrophy all exist and in none of them have we made any great progress for the prevention or cure. Metabolic diseases also include dental caries, and 98.5 per cent of our people, including the children, have dental caries. It, too, is a metabolic disease, caused primarily by malnutrition and poisons.

If this sounds dismal, let me sound an optimistic note. I think there is real hope left. We have time, if we get started on the right track and begin cleansing out the poisons from every link of the food chain and restore this country to proper nutrition. We can prevent this biological blight. We can save this nation from metabolic disaster.

I think we must learn to prevent cancer. We must learn to prevent heart disease in the old as well as the young. We must learn to prevent arthritis. We must learn to prevent birth defects.

We can prevent children's tragic deaths by the thousands. We live in a polluted world today, and I don't say that natural, poison-free food will bring in the millenium with perfect health free of disease, but it will do much of the job. I don't promise to abolish death; I do propose to postpone it for millions of persons, and one of those persons might be you, and your children.

If we continue to eat as we have been, as a nation, we will continue to have high incidences of metabolic diseases—even if wd had a pollution-free world.

In the past, physicians have said there is nothing basically wrong with the modern American food supply. A professor of nutrition at Harvard University has said, in effect, "Go into any grocery store and get a variety of the four food groups and you will get a proper, balanced diet." Well, I did this. It almost killed me. I got heart disease. Although poor nutrition is not the only cause of metabolic disease, it is by far the greatest cause.

There is a second point of view that has been espoused through the years. It is to continue eating these typical foods but to take, in addition, enough vitamins, minerals, and enzymes to ensure proper nutrition. This is the method of millions of Americans, and it is an improvement over the other. But I don't think it will prevent metabolic disease.

The third way is to eat natural, poison-free food grown on fertile soil, fresh and not overcooked. This is the ideal. For the majority of people in America at the present time, the ideal may be impossible. There is not enough natural, poison-free food available for everyone. But there is enough for the educated minority, and the supply is increasing every day. Some day, hopefully not far in the future, there will be enough for everyone. Whether there is or not depends on you and me.

The purpose of this book is to show you, the reader, the ideal diet and to help you find good food. Even after you are charged with knowledge and have learned how to obtain your food, most of you will still have to take vitamin supplements when you travel. I do. You can't expect to find, yet, natural food in our nation's restaurants and cafes. Therefore, there is a tremendous need for natural vitamins and mineral supplements today.

You and I will be the ones who will decide which road America will take in the years ahead. I, as a member of my generation, feel as personally responsible as anyone else for the state of our health. As a doctor, I feel responsible for my patients. As a father, I feel responsible not only for my children but for my grandchildren as well. My generation has despoiled this planet. My generation has permitted the poisons to go into our food. My generation—and perhaps yours, too—has permitted the overprocessing of foods so that the masses of America today are malnourished and this, we know, is one of the causes of mental retardation and birth defects. My generation and yours have permitted the widespread use of food additives that are known to cause cancer.

The answer to our metabolic disaster is simple: proper nutrition from natural foods. The ways we will arrive at that simple answer will not always be so simple. It may take long years before this nation is firmly set upon the new, shining road to health.

III.

A Concept of Totality

Visualize this scene. It is a dark wintry night in one of our great cities, and a man is walking down a lonely street. Snow is falling. Because it is cold, he is clothed completely, from his topcoat down to heavy socks, underwear, muffler, and gloves.

Suddenly, out of the shadows of an alley an armed man appears and points a .38 revolver at the head of our friend.

The accoster perfunctorily pockets our friend's wallet and watch, and then orders him to disrobe.

There is no choice but to obey. Soon our friend is stripped bare, his clothes in a heap on the snowy sidewalk. You can imagine how he feels, naked and shivering.

Then, as if suddenly suffused with generosity, the pistol-wielder tells our friend that, after all, it *is* a bit cold out tonight and he's going to do a great favor for him. He is going to give him some clothes for warmth. Down deep, it seems, he is a humanitarian.

So the gunman says, "Here, I'm going to make you richer and warmer."

He reaches into a bag he is carrying and gives our friend not any of the clothes he was stripped of, but an old tie and a hat and a synthetic sock with a hole in the toe for a left foot. The tie is outlandish and hardly a symbol of warmth, and the hat doesn't fit. But never mind. The gunman has given it to his victim, and he feels the recipient should be grateful.

Was our friend "enriched"—or was he robbed?

I am using this parable, if I may call it that, because it describes vividly, to me, what happens to a grain of wheat from the time it is harvested until it has entered a loaf of our American commercial white bread. The advertising term used to sell bread is *enrichment*. Let us see whether, indeed, it is enrichment—or robbery.

In the milling of white flour, the wheat germ and the outside layers of the grain are removed. This means that enzymes, vitamins, and minerals are stripped from the whole wheat grain in much the same way that our friend was stripped of his clothing during his winter night's stroll. Most of the vitamins and minerals are removed.

In combination with this stripping process used by the millers, for thirty years white flour was bleached with nitrogen trichloride, the agene process. This is a poison affecting the central nervous system. It gives puppies fits, and it may be one of the reasons why 50 per cent of the hospital beds in America are filled with mental patients.

However, on October 1, 1949, most of the millers voluntarily changed to the chlorine dioxide process of bleaching this vital foodstuff. But chlorine dioxide is also a poison. Its safety has not been proved!

Now, we have our grain of wheat in approximately the same predicament as our terrorized friend at the end of the dark alley. The grain of wheat has been stripped bare of everything that could be taken from it. In addition, it has been bleached by poison —comparable to our friend's having been shot or shot at.

At this point, after vital nutrients have been taken from the grain of wheat it is, to use the advertising term we have heard so often, *enriched*. This, we are being constantly told over the radio and television, and in the press, is a very scientific achievement that has made our daily bread such a valuable food.

But what is enriched bread? First, the processors take a perfectly good grain of wheat and then remove most of the vitamins and minerals. Then they start with raw starch. Into the raw starch they put back three little dead synthetic chemicals—niacin, thiamine, and riboflavin, plus inorganic iron. These three synthetic vitamins are a part of the vitamin B complex. But natural B complex—and the wheat germ is one of its very best sources—contains a score of known parts, *besides the still unknown factors.*

The germ is also the richest source of natural vitamin E, which has been proved to be essential to a normal cardiovascular system. The germ also, no doubt, contains enzymes and vitamins as yet unnamed. All of these many essential nutrients are removed, and only three synthetic vitamins plus a little iron are added.

This could hardly be accepted as enrichment. We call this fragmentation. Anytime there is fragmentation, we wind up with less than the whole we started with. Fragmentation may lead to peril, and it has, in fact, led to peril for consumers in this country in my lifetime.

A good analogy would be the creature that the medical student Frankenstein put together in his laboratory. A human being is a marvelous creation. Broken down into constituent parts, one can say a human being consists of a body functioning under full mental powers. There are bones, muscles, blood, tendons, organs. But the marvelous human body is the totality of all these, and because all these parts work in harmony, we have the human personality, which adds up to more than the sum of the parts. The important thing here is that the human body inevitably comes from a fertilized egg. It grows organically, or naturally, from that single cell. We do not produce human bodies in laboratories. There is only one way to do it. Dr. Frankenstein tried another way, by putting human parts together. This was a fragmented way of doing it—a quite unnatural way. Dr. Frankenstein wound up creating a monster. And you know what the monster did to him.

We have always thought of vitamin E as the reproductive vitamin, and it is essential to normal reproduction. Veterinarians have known this for seventy-five years and have fed pure wheat germ oil to the barren heifer and to the bulls with good results. This has been further demonstrated with other animals. Pregnant rats will abort on the thirteenth day every time if all the vitamin E is removed from the diet. Since 80 per cent of the food Americans eat has had all the life taken from it, it is no wonder that we have problems of sterility in our young women.

Although I have been speaking specifically of the damage that processing does to whole wheat, and its consequent loss of the valuable vitamin E, the situation is the same for other foods and especially so for the other grain foods. The ordinary store-bought cornmeal is worthless. It has been degerminated. This is supposed to improve its keeping quality, and it does. It keeps the weevils out. It also keeps me out. If a sack of meal is not good enough for a weevil, I doubt that it is good enough for a man.

Natural rice is one of the best foods in the world. Many people in the Orient live on it almost totally. It is one of the richest sources of natural vitamin B complex, which is essential to good health. But when we come to white rice, which is generally what we get in the United States, we are back to the old story of our friend who was robbed while walking down the street. White rice is exactly like natural rice—except that most of the vitamins and minerals have been polished away. And, again, this has been done for one reason only, and that reason has nothing at all to do with good health—just so the rice will keep in 100-pound bags and can be stored until it can be sold for a profit. In fact, health factors are not even considered in the processing and marketing stages. What is packaged and sold in grocery stores is not rice, as a matter of fact. Rice is a whole food, a natural food, and it contains all the factors it had when it was harvested. The rice that is so highly advertised and so gaily packaged is, in fact, raw starch—an item already superfluous to the high-carbohydrate American diet. The raw starch of white, polished rice is, in my opinion, unfit for human consumption.

Although we shall go into it in more detail later on in this book, I wish to mention briefly white sugar. White sugar fits in perfectly with white rice and white bread. They are buddies. White sugar is the worst food in the American diet. I have stated innumerable times, "It is so sorry that not even a worm will eat it." The fact is that white sugar is one of our most dangerous food items in this country. And again we come full circle as we did with the grain foodstuffs. Why is all the good part of the sugar removed—the molasses and the vitamins and minerals? Why are we left with nothing but carbohydrates and calories, which we have too much of already? It is done for a purely selfish commercial reason: so that the sugar will keep. Shelf, or storage, life. White sugar can be stored in 100-pound cloth sacks for years in dirty warehouses and still be sold for a profit. Where have we heard that before? Love of money is not only the root of all evil, it is also the root of most of our disease.

Now, whole wheat flour is perhaps the most important of all foods, because most people eat bread three times a day, seven days a week. The whole wheat, or natural, flour has a positive value. It is, as the name implies, *whole.* All that nature put there is still there. I am not referring to some brands of bread that are called whole wheat and, in fact, are not. Often these loaves have been processed to varying extents; almost always they have been enriched; often coloring has been added to make them look brown like whole wheat. The way to find out whether it's the real McCoy or not is to read the label carefully, the fine print, the works. Labels, fine print and all, tell a great deal about any product. The chances are, too, that if the print is fine, then there's something that somebody is trying to hide. It is almost a rule of thumb that producers of foods that aren't overprocessed are so proud of that fact that they proclaim it in large letters on the product, while those trying to hide something use fine print that is easy to overlook and hard to read.

This, then, is the positive value of the whole grain, or of any food that hasn't been overprocessed. It has all the vitamins, minerals, and enzymes that nature put there. It is natural. It is unfragmented. Fragmentation is exactly what it means in the dictionary term. *Webster's New World Dictionary of the American Language* defines fragmentation as "a breaking into fragments," and *fragment* is "a part broken away from the whole; broken piece; a detached, isolated, or incomplete part."

Overprocessed food is fragmented food. Just as the dictionary says, it is incomplete. Fragmented, or incomplete, food leads to incomplete nutrition. Incomplete nutrition leads to a nation of fat, sick people. That's what we have in America today.

I tell all my patients that they should *never buy any food that has been enriched.* If a food is so incomplete, or so sorry, to start with that synthetic chemical vitamins have to be added, then it is not worth their—or your—money. If you follow this rule, you automatically remove about 90 per cent of the breakfast foods from your diet, and this is a wise decision. They are no good. If they were, the bugs would get into them through the flimsy pasteboard boxes they come in, while sitting around the warehouses. Moreover, they are bad for you.

Fifty per cent of the calories that the average American eats comes from three things: white flour, white sugar, and hydrogenated fats. By hydrogenated fats, I refer primarily to compound shortenings and oleomargarine. Not one of these, in my opinion, is fit to eat.

Oleomargarine has been fortified with 15,000 units of vitamin A. That is one reason I think it is no good. Butter does not have to be fortified. But worse than that, hydrogenated fats have been tampered with fundamentally, more than most persons realize. The food processor found out that his oils and fats in their natural state would spoil and become rancid in time. This cost him money. But he discovered that if he added nickel for a catalyst and heated it under pressure, then he could force in hydrogen in four spots in the molecules. Once saturated with hydrogen, it became a saturated, or hydrogenated, fat that wouldn't spoil. This gave the food processor what he wanted most of all—shelf life. But unfortunately when he did this he destroyed the essential fatty acids. Note that I said *essential.* You've got to have them. I consider hydrogenated fats—which are found also in mellorine, store-bought peanut butter, cookies and breads, crackers, and practically all commercial bakery products—to be the Number One cause of heart disease. We have swapped our health for the processors' economic scheme, a poor exchange. In the end, shelf life spells food death.

I doubt that we will ever see a significant decrease in degenerative disease until the day comes when mothers can have natural food grown on fertile soil and then nurse their babies at the breast as nature provided and intended. Then, and only then, we will have a totally natural food supply that we can depend on.

Natural food? Fertile soil? We are coming again to the search I was involved in earlier. Natural food and fertile soil play vital, absolutely essential roles in our struggle to prevent fragmentation, or incomplete nutrition.

I call it "a concept of totality." All, or the whole, is essential. This implies balance. It is a philosophy, perhaps, but it is a fact of life—a law—we must obey, regardless of whether we call it a philosophy, a religious tenet, pragmatism, or just good, plain old common sense.

My concept of totality involves, of course, much more than merely consuming the whole grain product and natural oils and fats. It is a working arrangement—a balanced working arrangement—between man and nature. Man now recognizes there are natural laws he must obey or suffer the consequences. He cannot defy the law of gravity. If he walked out a twentieth-floor window, his attempt to defy the law of gravity would most likely result in his death. By the same token, man must also accept the equally binding rules of his working arrangement with nature.

He is part of the ecology, and he is not always as important a part of it as he would sometimes like to think.

Let us look a little deeper into the totality that man has been guilty of fragmenting. Let us begin where all food begins, or should begin—the soil.

It is literally true that good health is built from the ground up. The soil grows our food. We must start with fertile soil, or we have started with one strike against us. Of course we can spoil good food grown on fertile soil by overprocessing it. But if we do not start with fertile soil, we *start off* fragmented.

America is ravaged today by degenerative diseases. Yet there are places in the world where the degenerative diseases I mentioned earlier do not occur. In Hunza, near India, Sir Robert McCarrison, the British physician whose book helped change my life, stayed seven years. He looked for an instance of cancer without success during that time. These people live to be 110 years of age and die with their own teeth in their mouths! Seventy-year-old men run twenty miles a day and think nothing of it. These facts are so astounding to the modern American mind that perhaps I should repeat them.

Hunzas live to be 110 years of age and die with their own teeth in their mouths! Seventy-year-old men run twenty miles a day and think nothing of it.

A far cry from the America we know today? Yes, certainly.

How do the Hunzas do it? Well, Sir Robert said the reason these people have such excellent health is that they do two very simple things that we fail to do. They eat natural food grown on fertile soil, and they eat it fresh. We do neither of these.

Briefly, I would like to sketch for you what we have done in this country, and what is happening in other countries today.

Essentially, we have fragmented, or violated the totality of, nature. We have done to the soil what the profit-grasping flour manufacturer has done to the whole wheat grain. In doing so, the farmers of America have attempted to violate what I call Nature's Law of Return. It is the first great fundamental reason why all of us are sick, from the standpoint of nutrition—because the land is worn out. Nature's Law of Return states that if you take something from me, then you must return something of equal value to me or you will pay for it in some way. Our agricultural industry has attempted to violate this. I say *attempted,* because it cannot be violated, and the attempt to do so triggers sure consequences. How did the farmers attempt to violate it? They cut down the trees, plowed up the land, planted cotton one year and corn the next, and even burned the stalks. Constantly they, or we, if you wish, took out and never put anything back. ·

As a result, all the land became poor land. Poor land grows poor food that produces poor, sick people. Poor land grows food that is poor in vitamins, poor in minerals, poor in enzymes, and produces proteins of poor quality. All this spells poor health. Worn-out land has also been a basic cause of our people leaving the farms. Because they could not make a living on the land, they were forced to move into the ghettoes and slums of the big cities.

The most common disease in America today is hypoproteinemia. This is insufficient protein, or protein of poor quality, and it is of tremendous significance. The enzymes and the antibodies, which gives us resistance to disease, are all protein substances. If the soil is worn out and does not have this protein-producing capacity in the first place, how is it going to miraculously appear in the food? Where else but in food are we to get our protein supply?

About the time all the land became worn out, along came Science, completely capitalized and enshrined, to the rescue. In this country we have been conditioned to worship the word *science*. In this instance, the Great God Science, through the chemical trust that had convinced the U.S. Department of Agriculture, the A&M colleges, and the county agents, sold the farmers on commercial fertilizer. NKP, or nitrogen-potash-phosphate, became the godsend of Science to rescue the worn-out land.

The farmer was told, "If you will put this NKP on your land, we promise it will grow twice as much, and it will put money in the bank." Of course this was true. The land did produce twice as much. The farmer did put more money into the bank.

The millenium was here. NKP had saved the day—for the commercial fertilizer manufacturer. And the promises were true —for a while. But, as the years stretched on, the farmer learned that his land required more and more fertilizer, yet he got less and less in return. Nature's Law of Return was being demonstrated. NKP does not make land rich. It provides for quick growth of an inferior plant. It further destroys what remaining fertility is left in a worn-out soil. One of the reasons for this is that NKP is treated with acid that kills biotic life in the soil, such as earthworms and micro-organisms. Finally, as farmers have been discovering over the years, there is no living soil left. It is dead.

The end result of chemical farming is always disease. Disease comes first to the land itself, then to the plant, then in the animal, and finally to us, who eat the plants and the animals or their products. Everywhere in the world where chemical farming is widely practiced, the people are sick. Rather than make anything rich but the manufacturers, synthetic fertilizers make the land poorer than before.

There is one way and only one way to make land rich. That is the same method that nature uses on the forest floor. Nature does it perfectly, and we need to learn how by cooperating with nature rather than fighting nature as if *Homo sapiens* were in a war with the land—a struggle to the finish, one sometimes suspects. On the forest floor, dead plant matter and dead animal matter go back into the land. Leaf mold, through decay, gives continued life to the land. All together, these put everything back into the soil: the major elements, plus the trace elements, plus dead and decaying organic matter, and all in proper proportions. A careful study of the soil nutrients found on the forest floor, compared to fields doused with NKP, would cause any thinking person to uproariously chortle at the claim that NKP could possibly give to the land even a portion of what nature does.

Dead and decaying matter. This is a key phrase in understanding nature's fertilizers. *Dead and decaying matter* tells us that the material had life at one time. This is of tremendous importance. The leaf we spoke of is now leaf mold, slowly disintegrating, slowly returning to the soil from which the tree took the nutrients with which it made the leaf. The leaf was a living thing at one time. *You must have death and decay if you expect to have life and growth.* This is a natural cycle that no chemist can get around, no matter how many degrees he may have behind his name.

The end result of the decaying process is the amino acids and other organic acids. The amino acids are the little building blocks that the plants use to make protein of high quality. How can a plant manufacture proteins of high quality when it had no amino acids in the beginning? It cannot. You cannot make something out of nothing, nor can a plant. NKP cannot produce proteins of high quality, because it does not feed these essentials into the soil and thence to the plant. This is one of the fundamental reasons why the proteins produced on the farms of America are of such poor quality.

Fertile soil is usually dark in color. It is soft. When it rains, the water soaks into the ground. Fertile soil is full of both life and death—death and decay of organic matter, and life in the form of bacteria, molds, and earthworms.

I believe that when we plant a seed in a piece of poor land and then surround it with NKP, we get a plant that is susceptible to disease. This plant produces diseased fruit and the good Lord sends the bugs to destroy it. This is the "survival of the fittest." The diseased plant falls victim to the bugs. The healthy plant wards off insects and survives. But man, in his presumed infinite wisdom, interferes with nature's solution to the problem by bringing in a "scientific" application of DDT, which kills the insects. Then what? Next, we eat the diseased plant and its residue of DDT or other pesticides.

No wonder we get sick!

The concept of totality, however, is only partially explained by my discussion of food and the soil, a subject we will be returning to in much more detail in subsequent chapters. Let us now look into six major causes of disease, which will give us a larger picture of this concept.

The chief causes of disease are:

1. Poisons.
2. Poor nutrition.
3. Emotional stress.
4. Infections.
5. Accidents.
6. Genetic.

We have discussed poor nutrition and how it fits into the concept of totality. Related to it are the poisons that in some form are introduced into the human system. We have touched upon this problem in our treatment of poor nutrition. Repeated applications of NKP in our soils eventually bring nitrates into our food chain, to our misfortune, as we shall see, later in this book. But the more dramatic way in which we are being poisoned is through the dumping of pesticides on our vegetables and in the raising of food animals. In the years since Rachel Carson first warned of pesticides in *Silent Spring*, use of DDT and other dangerous, long-lasting poisons has continued. Pesticides and pollution of every kind are daily bringing plagues of disease upon our populace. Sometimes poisons and poor nutrition are so closely interwoven that they are merely two sides of one coin. And their toll is taken in all ages and sexes of our people. Cancer, emphysema, heart disorders—these are but some of the better-known diseases that are caused by poisons in our food and in our environment and by poor nutrition.

Back in 1952, when I was formulating both a practical approach and a philosophy of health, I made an address to the Texas Bankers Association, which I called "A Concept of Totality." I was chairman of the board of my hometown Atlanta National Bank. Following the general theme of what I have just discussed in this chapter, that "Concept" did not go into such detail, and it did not contain all of the same material. Furthermore, when I discussed the six chief causes of disease, I did not rank them as I have here in this book.

At that time I rated emotional stress as the first leading cause of disease. It remains a major reason for disease, but in my opinion it is no longer Number One, but Number Three. Diseases, and causes of diseases, are subject to fluctuation just as are top-ranked college football teams!

In 1952 I stated, "The greatest cause of disease is, without a doubt, emotional stress. Worry, fear, anxiety, hate, envy, jealousy —these are the great killers. When any of these emotions takes hold of us, we get a conflict, and that conflict leads to tension."

This is still true. If you hate me, then I become a "pain in the neck" to you. The conflict causes tension on the muscles of the neck. At first there is a drawing in the back of the neck and, finally, if the conflict is intense enough, a tension headache results. The pain is not in the mind or the heart. It is in the back of the neck, right where the muscles join onto the head.

You have heard the expression, "I am fed up with that fellow." When you get angry at someone, then you are almost literally fed up with him. You get a full feeling in the stomach. The conflict causes tension and you get nervous indigestion. The expression probably arose from accumulated experience of many persons.

If the conflict is intense enough and is prolonged enough, and if some of the other factors of disease are present—especially, poor nutrition and poisons—then you get a peptic ulcer. We say that nervous indigestion is inorganic, or functional, but inorganic diseases are the forerunners of organic disease.

Heart disease is the leading cause of death in America today. How do these adverse emotions affect the heart? Simple. Conflict and tension cause the coronary vessels to constrict. The heart muscle itself does not get enough blood, and the heart cries out, so to speak, in pain. We call this symptom angina, which is functional or inorganic. This is what my heart condition was diagnosed as, in the absence of hard evidence of anything more critical. But if the conflict persists and if other factors of disease are present, then the patient gets coronary thrombosis.

All organic disease is made worse by emotional upset. I know a man who has gout. He gets along very well until he gets angry. Then he has to go to the hospital to have his gout treated.

What does one do about the emotional causes of disease? There are three things that can be done to resolve a conflict.

The first possibility is to run away from the conflict. If a husband comes home at three o'clock in the morning with lipstick on his shirt, his good wife is likely to get an emotional upset complete with headache, backache, indigestion, and heart pain. What can she do about it? Well, one solution would be for her to go back home to Mama. She could run away from the conflict.

A second solution would be to change the situation. She might become a better wife and cause the fellow to want to rush home at five o'clock with a clean shirt.

But there are some conflicts from which we cannot run away, and which we cannot change. If there is a death in the family, what can we do? What if the house burns to the ground? These conflicts must be *accepted,* if we are to remain healthy emotionally and mentally. There is no alternative.

Saying you accept a situation, however, is not the same as accepting it. It must be completely accepted, thought through both intellectually and emotionally, in order to end the conflict and tension. But few people really know how to accept these conflicts. This is done by knowing and practicing what I call the Three Great A's.

The first A is *Acceptance*—acceptance of the other fellow as an individual with rights and opinions of his own and also with his imperfections. There has been none perfect since Jesus, that I have heard of. If a wife expects her husband to be perfect at all times, she will be disappointed, and vice versa.

The second A is *Approval.* A pat on the back is much better than a kick in the pants. It's an old saying, even a cliche, but it's true. Things just work that way. Nor is the feeling of approval or disapproval communicated only by overt actions or words. It has been said that most of the conflict that arises between persons is caused by the *tone of voice* in which they speak. Approval can't be faked. If it isn't real, the other person will detect it on some level, possibly consciously, certainly unconsciously.

The third great A, and by far the most important one, I think, is *Adoration,* or love. This suggests what I call a great natural law, the Law of Love. No man can ever violate any natural law. This is the central idea of our concept of totality. Natural law is simple, self-evident, universal, and inviolate. You can jump from a fourteen-story building, but you do not violate the law of gravity. Your broken body is simply the exemplification of the law. I believe the law of love is a natural law and no man can violate it. Thus, the cure for the emotional cause of disease is very simple. All one has to do is to stop attempting to violate the law of love.

The law of love is divided into two parts: first, love God, and second, love thy neighbor. You cannot hate your neighbor and get by with it. He will become a pain in your neck. And it makes no difference how much he may have mistreated you, you still cannot afford to hate him. Worry, fear, and anxiety attempt to violate the first part of the law of love. The cure for the emotional cause of disease is to stop attempting to violate the law of love.

Thus, our concept of totality approaches healthful living from several directions. It is the only way to keep from fragmenting our lives. We must have emotional security and serenity to lessen the stress that can bring on disease by weakening our bodies. We must strengthen our bodies and minds by eating natural food grown on fertile soil, fresh and not overcooked or overprocessed.

For millions of years, the human body has been adjusting to its environment, just one part of the total ecology. During this time it has developed special needs. I think it can be stated that all but a few generations of these millions of years the human body has used as its fuel natural food. Over the millions of years our marvelous human body grew habituated to a food supply very much unlike our present-day highly processed and refined food. The body developed needs for specific enzymes. The digestive system became programmed to break down natural food, and this particular type of food had influences on the roles of the different organs. Diabetes, for instance, is a "civilized" disease and is directly related to white, or refined, sugar. We shall explore this later, but briefly we can state that white sugar and its by-products interfere with the role of the pancreas that has developed over the millions of years. Until relatively recently, the human pancreas dealt with natural sugars as they were found in plants or in honey. It performed this mission well. But with the introduction of white sugar in the diet, the pancreas—to cite just one effect—was unduly stressed and its natural processes short-circuited. The human body, accustomed and designed to use natural food as fuel, can't be expected to change within the space of even a few thousand years—much less five, ten, or twenty years—without becoming unduly stressed or diseased. We are doing much worse things to our more valuable human bodies than we are doing to our automobiles.

Can mankind afford this?

IV.

The Making of 'A Concept'

In the late 1940s and early 1950s I was, as I said in a preceding chapter, a "real, sure-nuff goin' joker" about natural foods. A zealot, perhaps. At the risk of my life I had seen the light and I was prepared to spread the news. I talked to farm groups, civic clubs, and churches. Although I had but one basic speech, I modified the title from one audience to the other. I might call it "Solomon's Secret" or perhaps "How to Live to Be a Hundred and Get Shot by a Jealous Husband and Still Go to Heaven." The latter formula for Heaven was not for church groups. I tried to add humor whenever possible, as in "The Virtues of a Fertile Egg." Just look at the hen that lays the commercial grocery-store egg, I would say; the poor old hen's been cooped up where she can't move around. She hasn't even seen a rooster, much less get caught by one! How can an unhappy hen lay a good egg? But under the surface I was deadly serious. I knew most of the eggs consumed by the American people were infertile, and this was strictly because there was more profit in an infertile egg. Again, profit rules over health. Stores pay more for infertile eggs because they keep longer, and for no other reason. God knows, they do not taste as good as a fertile egg, and I believe it is an attempt to violate natural law to keep the rooster off the chickenyard. The fertile egg has in it "life," whatever that is. It has a potentiality to bring forth another living thing. An infertile egg cannot do this. There obviously is a biological difference, and this difference is translated into a nutritional advantage that the infertile egg does not have.

When I talked with drug salesmen and other skeptics, I did a presentation I called "Solomon's Secret." To get their attention, I explained that I had done research on the Bible. This elicited only mild response. Then I mentioned that Soloman had 700 wives and 300 concubines and that it had been rumored he had seduced the Queen of Sheba. That did it, every time. They sat up, ears straining and absorbing like blotters. Yeah, they seemed to say, tell us about ol' Solomon! What *was* his secret?

Then I explained how Solomon, back in Biblical times, was eating the whole wheat product, thereby getting his full quota of vitamin E, among other essential vitamins, minerals, and enzymes. Although vitamin E is essential to good heart action and as a conservator of oxygen it is very significant to good circulation, its public image is more related to its role as a "sex vitamin." Vitamin E, which is found abundantly in the whole wheat grain, aids in conception from both the male and female sides of the picture.

During this time, while I was searching for an effective means of communication for the natural food story, I was also developing my personal approach to health. Out of my heart problem, my own "concept of totality" was growing.

Perhaps more accurately, my concept of totality had been growing all my life. The heart problem and the events following it gave substance and shape to my life and thoughts. This period was my crucible. But upon coming out of the crucible I could see more clearly the events of my life before that point, and I understood them as I never had before.

In many ways, the story of my ancestors and my own life history parallels the story of this nation of ours. It tells a lot about the health of this country and for that reason I would like to give some details from my own personal background.

My Great-great-grandfather Nichols owned a big plantation in South Carolina, where he cleared the land and planted cotton, corn, and tobacco. The land was rich, the cost of labor cheap, and he was industrious and a good manager. With adequate rainfall, the fertile virgin soil grew crops in abundance, with healthy plants, which meant there was no insect problem. Consequently, he made lots of money. He built a big house and educated a large family. He had, it seemed, found the land of milk and honey.

Unfortunately, he knew little about conservation. Year after year the planter took big yields from the fertile soil. But he put nothing back. As I came to realize later, he was attempting to violate the Law of Return. Gradually, as the once-fertile soils lost their organic content and biotic life, the yields became smaller. Then he simply cleared more land and continued the exploitation.

Finally, there was no more land to be cleared. The family fortune began to decline. By the time my Great-grandfather Nichols was grown, the plantation was exhausted. So he, the son, had to move. He took Horace Greeley's advice and went west, to Tennessee, seeking a new start. There, which was "out West" then, he got 2,000 acres of very fertile soil. He cleared the land and grew cotton, corn, and tobacco. He was an energetic, husky man who stood six-feet-six and weighed 350 pounds, and he worked hard, led a good life, and enjoyed good health. He made money, built a big house, and educated a large family.

The topsoil was his greatest natural resource. From it had come his wealth, health, and his ability to educate his children. But, again, he had not learned the lesson of conservation. He destroyed the fertility of his land the same way his father had done in South Carolina. In less than a generation, his Tennessee farm was ruined.

When his son William Nichols—my grandfather—was grown, he moved to Alabama, also seeking new land and new opportunity. This was the frontier American way of doing things: exploit the land until it was exhausted and then move on to new, virgin earth. Land was considered practically limitless in those days; moving on was a way of life. My grandfather, William Nichols, bought 2,000 acres of fertile soil and virgin timber on Horse Creek in Maringo County, Alabama, about fifty miles south of the beautiful old city of Selma. Like his ancestors, he made money, built a big house, and had twelve children. He even established a little town called Nicholsville where he owned a sawmill, a general store, and a grist mill. He fought in the Civil War and ate shoe leather—perhaps a natural food of sorts, but overprocessed—at the siege of Vicksburg to survive. His was a healthy family. He always had a garden with fresh, poison-free vegetables and animals that provided poison-free meats and eggs, raw milk and butter. Cancer in those days was a rare disease, found only in the very old.

William Nichols was not a greedy or selfish man. In fact, he was a Bible student, a leader in the Baptist Church, and a genuinely good man who gave generously to civic and religious causes. Yet in his ignorance of conservation practices of the topsoil he practiced a sort of subtle greed that eventually destroyed his farm. By then it was an old story, one repeated over and over across America, but it was one from which few, if any, had learned the significant lesson.

Thaddeus Lee Nichols, my father (named for General Robert E. Lee, whom my grandfather admired), was the last of my grandfather's twelve children, and he followed the family tradition of getting a good education. He graduated from Howard College in Birmingham, Alabama, with a major in mathematics. But most of the land around Nicholsville was depleted by that time, the people were sick, and he saw no future for him there. So he moved. He settled at Parkdale, Arkansas, a beautiful little town of about 300 on Bayou Bartholomew in Ashley County. In this rich Mississippi River delta country of Southeast Arkansas, my father started his business career as a bookkeeper in a general store. He worked long and hard, as had his ancestors, until he soon had his own store; then he bought 1,000 acres of good land on the bayou.

There were eight children in our family; two of them died in infancy. I was the second, coming fourteen months after my brother Lee, a fact I could use in later years to tease my mother about my being an unplanned child. (I also used to tease her about the unplanned birth of my youngest brother, T. K., who was born in the depression of the 1920s; T. K. now practices medicine with me.) My father had a big general store in Parkdale and we did a big "furnishing" business. The plantation owners would list the "bill of goods" required by the tenants every other Saturday. I worked in the store from the time I was nine years old, and I quickly learned how to fill orders. A typical order included flour, sugar, salt, lard, dry salt pork bellies, coffee, beans, snuff, and chewing tobacco. For medicine, they bought castor oil, Simmons Liver Regulator, and Tichenor's Antiseptic. They brought their own corn to town, and I swapped freshly ground cornmeal with them, bushel for bushel. On Fridays after school, I ground the corn on an old stone mill, and we fed our milk cows the rougher outside bran siftings. The corn was open-pollinated and of much greater nutritional value than today's hybrid corn.

My brothers and I milked the cows, so that we had plenty of good cold sweet milk, buttermilk, clabber, and butter. We also had a meat market inside the store, of locally killed meats. We sold patent medicines but had no pharmacy. In those days the doctors did not give much medicine. Quinine and calomel were standard remedies for malaria and "biliousness" so prevalent then. But cancer, diabetes, and heart disease were uncommon, and the same were almost unknown in children.

We did not stock many canned goods. Beans, peas, and even green coffee beans were sold in the bulk and were our staples. We bought flour by the carload and stored it in the back of the store where we also had a huge platform for the dry salt bellies.

The countryside abounded with quail, squirrels, coons, possums, and mink. People came to Ashley and Chicot Counties from miles around to hunt deer. The deer are still there in a few restricted areas, but the fish and much of the small game have been wiped out. The killer in this case was the pesticide DDT, which farmers sprayed on their cotton. DDT has been very successful on the wildlife, but it has failed on its stated target, the boll weevil, which continues its destructive ways.

In the family tradition, we all studied and worked to get a good education. I did not start to school until I was eight because of a serious eye problem diagnosed as trachoma. It required the treatment of a famed opthamologist in Little Rock, Arkansas, before I could attend classes. This doctor later because dean of the University of Arkansas Medical School. However, this eye problem was not allowed to hamper my learning. My mother taught me how to read and write and spell; my father taught me simple mathematics; I graduated from high school in Parkdale in 1924 at the age of fifteen.

I entered Ouachita Baptist College that fall, enrolling in a pre-medical course. I had decided to study medicine because I could see, already, that a successful farm operation was becoming more difficult. And looking back now, I can see the roots of many of our farming problems tracing to those days of the 1920s. My father was a civic and religious leader, and he had the reputation for being a progressive man. A "progressive" man heeded the discoveries and teachings of science, and my father was no exception. I remembered the times he would take a ferry across the Mississippi River at Greenville, Mississippi, and return with government bulletins extolling the virtues of commercial fertilizer and insecticides. My father, a good and educated man, believed the government bulletins contained scientific truth about better farming methods. He thought he was doing something good for the country when he bought the first carload of fertilizer in our area. Before long, everybody else was using it on his farm too. As predicted, production of some crops doubled. But the insect population doubled too. The boll weevil became a threat to the cotton crop. It previously had not caused much trouble. And a new threat to the cotton crop, the leaf hopper, appeared.

The cotton crop of 1926 is memorable to me. By then the government research station at Starkville, Mississippi, had another bulletin describing an insecticide that would eradicate the insects and save the cotton. Of course, the cost of production had gone up and the farmer could never be sure about the price of cotton. That summer my brother Lee and I had finished the sophomore year at Ouachita, and we went home to work on the farm. We had fifty acres of cotton planted on the best piece of land left, and we had a good stand. At 4:30 every morning we were out of bed and headed for the big barn in our old Ford truck and by sun-up we were in the field plowing a pair of good young mules and a cultivator. My father had used plenty of fertilizer, and we had a bumper crop. We had bugs too, but we stayed up nights dusting on an insecticide that required the dew to stick to the cotton plant and get the bugs.

I worked harder that summer than I ever had before or have since. We made two bales on every acre, an excellent yield. Everybody made a lot of cotton in 1926. When Lee and I left for our junior year of college in September, the fields were white with cotton.

When we came home for the Christmas vacation, the fields were still white with cotton. The price had gone to nine cents per pound that fall. The bumper crop of cotton wasn't worth picking. And I was surer than ever that I wanted to study medicine.

I wish I could say my diet was a sensible one then, but I can't. At Ouachita Baptist College, I held a basketball scholarship and because of it I got the job of looking after the milk, which came in five-gallon cans. It was good raw milk and the basketball players got the cream, but some of our other food was not so good. I ate white sugar, white bread, refined salt, and the other convenience foods that today I know cause heart disease. I weighed 186 pounds when I graduated and although all this contributed to my subsequent heart problem in 1946, it was nothing new to my diet. I had eaten the same junk foods out of our store in Parkdale, although I also got some protective foods from our garden and the farm. We didn't know much about nutrition. My father also ate the same junk foods from our store. He had a stroke when he was sixty. At sixty-three, he was dead of a heart attack.

I entered the University of Arkansas Medical School in 1928. Although nobody had much money in those days, so that it was a financial strain to get through medical school, in other ways it was an excellent time to study medicine. People were sick as well as poor. Doctors were needed urgently. I shared a third-floor back bedroom with another struggling medical student for $10 a month, four blocks from the school, and we found a boarding house that served "good" food for 35 cents a meal, and we were ready to get an education.

Our first interview was with the assistant professor of anatomy. He was in his seventies and had taught anatomy to medical students for years. He looked over the class and spotted the brilliant ones. I was not in that group. I will never forget the sound advice he gave. He said, "Some of you have come here with brilliant records in college. Some of you are intellectuals. Some of you think that you can breeze through medical school just like you breezed through high school and college. But I have news for you. The only way you can pass my course in anatomy at this medical school is by a short four-letter word. You spell it W-O-R-K. You hope to become a doctor of medicine. If you do, you will hold the difference between life and death in your hands. You must know basic anatomy of the human body if you expect to pass this course. And unless you pass this course in anatomy, you will have to go back home and be a farmer or something else."

He gave us a box of human bones. He gave us an assignment for the next day. He told us to know all about the long bone in the arm by the next morning. And he made me believe that he meant what he said!

As hard and challenging as my first year in medical school was, I no longer had any doubts about wanting to be a doctor. Perhaps the challenge was part of the attraction. Also, the Great Depression was on and there were no jobs anywhere, and nobody had any money. My uncle, Noble Daniel, was a junior in medical school, and he kept me both scared and encouraged. I soon knew

Sir William Osler was right. Medical school was an exacting taskmaster.

Unfortunately, the subject of proper nutrition was not taught at the University of Arkansas at that time. We took courses in biochemistry and learned how to write the structural formula for vitamin E and the female sex hormone, but we learned practically nothing about proper nutrition.

Through a number of jobs that included working the PBX board for an appliance company, a night shift at the YMCA, assistant librarian at the medical library, and selling microscopes for a doctor in downtown Little Rock, I financed my way through medical training. Soon my uncle, already Dr. Daniel, arranged for me to work as an extern at the Pulaski County Hospital during my junior year.

At the close of my sophomore year a great summer opportunity opened up that was to have a significant influence on my life. The professor of pathology, who was a close friend of Dan Beard at Flushing, Long Island, had always sent a student to Dan Beard's scout camp in the Poconos in Pennsylvania, as the camp doctor. The job was offered to a friend of mine, but he declined it and passed it on to me.

Dan Beard was a great conservationist and a founder of the Boy Scouts movement in America. He was one of the great naturalists of our time. If he were here today, DDT would have to go. I do not believe Dan Beard and DDT could occupy the same planet at the same time. Everybody respected and admired the Chief.

That fall I returned to medical school for my junior year, supporting myself with room and board at the old Pulaski County Hospital in Little Rock, signing insurance reports at 50 cents each, working in the venereal disease clinic, and finally selling my microscope for $150 to finish the year. And that summer I returned to Dan Beard's camp for another glorious season as camp doctor, a precedent-shattering repeat. By then I was more confident, as well, for I had done a half-dozen appendectomies at the Pulaski County Hospital and had circumcised dozens of boys from the detention home there.

In my senior year I got a job at the New Baptist Hospital as an extern assigned to the X-ray department. In 1932, in the depths of the Depression, I borrowed $300 from my cousin, Robin Nichols, and paid my back fees and graduated in style as a Doctor of Medicine. I was a very ambitious young doctor.

Another cousin, Harry Jackson, a surgeon in Birmingham, Alabama, persuaded me to go to Norwood Hospital there for my internship. It was a 200-bed private hospital owned by Dr. C. M. Carraway, with sixteen doctors in the clinic across the street. Dr. Carraway was one of the best surgeons in Birmingham, and the hospital stayed full most of the time. As an intern I was paid $50 a month and loved it. The other intern was in love and I was anxious to work and learn, so I was on call practically every night while he attended the object of his affections. We alternated every month on medicine and surgery. The clinic had three surgeons, and both of us assisted in the operating room every morning.

One morning in January, 1933, Dr. Carraway called me in and asked if I would go to a small mining town about twenty miles over the mountains. The flu epidemic had hit, and the doctor there was sick. The whole country was blanketed with snow; I barely made it over the mountain in a borrowed car. I learned much from that experience and much from the good doctor who was sick. For three days and nights I went up one street and down another, seeing the young and old who had flu and pneumonia. We had no antibiotics. We had a limited supply of codeine, which I dispensed very carefully. For the other cases I administered white aspirin, blue aspirin, pink aspirin, and, in the less severe illnesses, chalk tablets. The doctor had a large supply of chalk tablets. They worked wonders. That month the doctor taught me how to practice medicine without using much medicine, a lesson I have never forgotten. Proper rest, clean living habits, proper nutrition, and common sense in regard to emotional problems—these are often the most effective prescriptions a doctor can give.

A month later Dr. Carraway sent me to Leeds, Alabama, a town of about 2,000. Both the doctors there were sick. Leeds had three coal mines, a cement factory, a metal works factory, and three convict camps. The convicts were building a new highway through the mountains. Everybody had the flu. I stayed in Leeds for a month and worked eighteen hours or more every day and night. At one convict camp I had thirty patients in the "hospital," which was nothing more than a long, open-aired, cheaply-constructed building. Although many of them had pneumonia, all of them got well. They had plenty of fresh air, good food, and strong constitutions. Even though one of them had empyema he pulled through.

Late one afternoon I got a call to go over the mountain to deliver a baby. It was raining and the road was impossible. We walked a mile over the mountain to a little shack in the valley below where I attended a long and difficult first delivery. Every time the patient had a pain, her mother cried out. Finally I gave her a shot of morphine and sent her mother out of the house to await the results in the barn.

That left me alone with the laboring mother-to-be and an old Negro midwife who was just a little jealous of the new doctor.

Finally the midwife said, "You sho do look young to be a doctor."

I was only twenty-four years old. Soon afterward I grew a mustache.

Dr. Carraway invited me to remain as a member of his clinic after my internship, and I looked forward to a good life in Birmingham, but events dictated otherwise. On July 1, 1933, the day I completed my internship, a telegram arrived from Dr. Daniel, my uncle, who was practicing medicine in Texarkana, Texas. He had fallen down an open elevator shaft. He had fractured his ankle, and he was without money or insurance, in the midst of the Depression, with a wife and a small son to support. Could I come to take care of his practice until he was on his feet again?

There was only one answer I could give. During the depression of 1921 when my father was ill, Dr. Daniel had given up a good job to go to Parkdale and take care of my father's business. When I showed the telegram to Dr. Carraway, he agreed my place was in Texarkana.

When I arrived there, Dr. Daniel said, "Joe, that's the *worst* broken leg I ever saw!"

I had seen the X-ray and I replied, "Oh, Dan, I've seen lots of 'em worse."

"Yeah," he said, "but that's *my* leg."

Six months later, Dr. Daniel was off crutches and together we moved into a refurnished office in a bank building. By then things were going well. Then one day H. H. Ramsey, a friend of Dr. Daniel, came to see us. He came from Atlanta, Texas, a little town about twenty miles from Texarkana. Atlanta was desperately in need of a young doctor. Its three doctors were older and not in good health. It was difficult to get a doctor at night.

Dr. Daniel and I drove to look over the beautiful little town. It was filled with friendly people. It was obvious that Atlanta was a town with a future that would attract some young doctor quickly. I loved Atlanta from the first day—November 23, 1933. Dr. Daniel gave me an old black bag, a stethoscope, a blood pressure machine, and a $5 bill. A local druggist took me to my new home and curtained off a corner of his drugstore for an office. I bought a used red Chevrolet coupe for $250 with nothing down, and I was in business.

On my first day in Atlanta, a little girl came in with a bean in her ear. The bean had been there for two days and was swollen. I didn't have an instrument capable of extracting the bean. But the dentist upstairs did. That day I performed one of the most difficult operations I had faced. Later that same day a salesman came calling from a surgical supply house in Shreveport, Louisiana, and made the easiest sale of his career. He took me to Shreveport and sold me $500 worth of instruments, on credit.

This was 1933, in the depths of the Great Depression, and Cass County was one of the poorest of the 254 counties in Texas. Yet in six months I was making more money than the president of the local bank, who had been there a lifetime—even though my office visits did not average over 50 cents each and house calls weren't over one dollar! But all the land was poor and all the people were sick, and I had *volume.*

The story of Cass County dovetails neatly with my ancestors' stories that I have already told you. The county was settled about 1850, primarily by people leaving the worn-out farms in the vicinity of Atlanta, Georgia. Place names like Douglassville, Marietta, and Smyrna are found near both Atlantas. In East Texas these people made the same mistakes their parents had made in Georgia. They mined the soil. They planted cotton one year and corn the next. As soon as they learned of the great virtues of commercial fertilizer, they proceeded with vigor to exploit the land.

Average annual rainfall in Cass County is 50 inches a year. Originally, the area was covered with pine trees. The topsoil was composed of clay and iron ore gravel. There never was much organic matter on most of the land. A pine tree does not require much organic matter to survive. It only produces cellulose. You do not go squirrel hunting in a pine forest. But the Cass County countryside also has a rolling terrain, and the Sulphur River and creek bottoms did grow oak and hickory trees that produced nuts rich in protein. So squirrel hunting was good in the bottoms. But much of the topsoil had washed off the overcultivated hills and had vanished down the Red River and into the mighty Mississippi. The land was poor, the people were poor, and they were sick.

I had a ready-made practice. Most of the 30,000 Cass Countians were either sick or thought they were sick. I saw from 50 to 100 patients per day, including Sundays. But all weren't sick. Some were merely pregnant. I delivered an average of 30 babies a month, all in the homes. There was no hospital there then. In one 24-hour period I delivered three sets of twins, two of whom bear my first name in recognition of my efforts.

Paradoxically, I made my money when there was no money, in the Depression. But I worked hard for it and I never let up. In the spring of 1935, having persuaded Dr. Ernest Grumbles, an old friend of mine, to join me, we opened up our own clinic. Three months later oil was discovered in Rodessa, Louisiana, only fifteen miles away. The oil operators were in a hurry to get the oil out of the ground and safety standards were poor, and they had an "epidemic of accidents" that kept our clinic even busier. In addition, oil workers would stop at the taverns in wet Louisiana before returning to dry Texas. There was a sharp curve between the state line and Atlanta. Traffic injuries climbed sharply.

Having to refer the more serious cases to Texarkana or Shreveport, we soon saw the need for a hospital in Atlanta. Dr. Grumbles and I explored the possibility. The City of Atlanta gave us the land, and after getting the necessary loan we had a modern 12-bed hospital and clinic built. A week after it opened in June, 1936, it was filled, and it has been since. Today we have six doctors and it has been expanded to 35 beds.

I loved being busy. I served as president of the Chamber of Commerce, the Rotary Club, and when World War II came I became chairman of the Red Cross and the USO. The strain during the war was even greater, for we were trying to operate a hospital with little help. Atlanta by then had grown, and we had a scarcity of doctors both in town and in the county.

Having joined the local medical society, I became very active in organized medicine. I became a delegate to the Texas Medical Association, where I served for twenty years. I also served nine years on the TMA Board of Councilors, which may be compared to the Supreme Court's role in our federal government.

This was the personal heritage I had behind me on May 23, 1946, when I suffered my heart seizure—and slowly began my struggle back to health.

By 1950 I was busily making speeches on whole wheat and fertile eggs and organic farming generally, and by then I had developed a personal philosophy of health that I thought important enough to share with others. And how I shared it! I rarely missed an opportunity.

One day in Dallas where I was attending a bankers convention (I was chairman of the board of my bank, by then), my wife Mildred and I were walking down a corridor at the Baker Hotel.

Nodding toward the man ahead of us, she whispered to me, "I know him. He used to go with my twin sister Mina at SMU."

We went up to him and Mildred said, "Hello there; I think I know you."

"Why, hello there, Mina," he said.

"You still can't tell us apart!" she said, laughing.

He introduced his wife and after talking a while we planned to dine together the next evening at the Dallas Country Club. At that time I told him some of my stories. One of them was "Solomon's Secret." This was in March, 1951.

The next week I had a letter from him. He was chairman of the program committee of the Texas Bankers Conference, which was having a Labor Day weekend meeting at the University of Texas in Austin. It was to be an intensive three-day conference for young bankers. He thought I had some humor that would hold their attention and keep them on campus. He wanted me to make a speech on Sunday night.

I gave a presentation similar to "Solomon's Secret." I drew a picture of a grain of wheat and explained the great virtues of vitamin E, the reproductive vitamin. The best source of it was wheat germ, I told them. Since then my friends in banking circles have called me "Wheat Germ" Nichols.

That speech led to another, more important one. That weekend I was invited to make the same speech to the annual Texas Bankers State Convention in Galveston in May, 1952. I accepted the invitation immediately. Making speeches had become my major form of recreation.

A month or so before I was to make the speech, I had a letter from William Philpott, Jr., executive secretary of the Texas Bankers Association. He wanted a copy of the speech. I didn't have one, nor had I expected to write one. All my speeches were extemporaneous. But he insisted that I write it down for his inspection before delivery. Bankers are a cautious lot. He was no exception.

"Dr. Nichols," he said, "I've got to know more about the speech. I've got to know what you are going to say."

So one Sunday afternoon I wrote the speech. It concentrated on all the factors that go into disease. We cannot violate the laws of nature. I included the law of love as one of these. This had been pointed up dramatically to me one day after my heart problem when I had picked up the local weekly, the Atlanta *Citizens Journal,* and had seen the picture of a person I had had troubles with. Looking at him, and reliving the emotions I felt toward him, I had the most severe attack of angina, or heart pain, I had ever had. It convinced me never again to harbor any thoughts of dislike toward another person. It is sensible and practical for physiological reasons as well as others, for tension causes the heart to constrict, thereby limiting its supply of oxygen. It pays to love your neighbor.

All my beliefs about living in harmony with natural law were incorporated into that concept. At that time I wrote that emotional causes of disease were the number one cause. Although worry, fear, anviety, hate, envy, and jealousy all do make you sick, I have since revised my thinking to place malnutrition and poisons as the chief causes of disease. Today there is more poisoning, more malnutrition, and less resistance to disease. Poisons are destroying enzymes in our bodies, and even if we eat good foods and have too much of these poisons entering our bodies, we will kill those enzymes.

I hadn't named my speech yet. That came during a vacation in Colorado. I had a dream and woke up that morning and the title was there. I called it "A Concept of Totality."

In May, 1952, I delivered the speech as scheduled. Philpott wanted to pay me $250 for the speech, but I refused to take any money. I had met some traveling nutritionists in California and other places who were paid lecturers. Some of them had "magic products" to sell. I didn't want to be put into the same category with them. I didn't want to get branded as one who was making money on the basis of unorthodox views. I had nothing to sell but an idea, and it was free. I had benefitted, and I wanted to share what I had discovered.

But Philpott persisted. He printed my speech in the *Texas Bankers Record,* and he insisted that I accept 10,000 reprints of the article. This I did, without further argument, and I began a new campaign, a giveaway educational journey through the printed word. It was a significant turn in my life.

Everywhere I went I gave away reprints of "A Concept of Totality." I left them behind in motels, hotels, filling stations, restaurants, everywhere I made speeches. Since then the "Concept" has been found in the most unusual places. A mining engineer in Peru found a copy in an old mine and wrote me for another one. A Texas friend of mine, Josh Morriss, Sr., found one under his bed at the Waldorf Astoria Hotel in New York. The "Concept" has now been translated into Danish, Finnish, French, Korean, Spanish, German, and Japanese. It has been scattered to the four winds.

V.

NFA—An Idea Becomes Flesh

Late one night in 1952, while I was attending a medical convention in Houston, I had a long distance call from a man who had been trying to get in touch with me all day. First he had called my home. My wife had referred him to my hotel in Houston.

"Dr. Joe Nichols?" said the man on the other end of the phone.

"Yes."

"I'm Dr. Fred Miller of Altoona, Pennsylvania," he said. "I'm a dentist and you never heard of me. I've read your 'Concept of Totality' and I like it, and I want one thousand copies."

"Dr. Miller, I don't have that many left. I've just got two hundred."

"Well, send me half of those and I'll pay for them."

"I'll send them to you and it won't cost you anything," I said.

What did he want with 1,000 copies? This great dentist and nutritionist was a kindred soul. He was going to scatter them, give them to patients, to anyone who would read them. Dr. Miller was, and is, dedicated to the pursuit of sound nutrition and good health. His book, *Open Door to Health* (Devin-Adair, N.Y., 1959), should be compulsory reading for every dental and medical student in the country, whether he is still at the university or a graduate. Furthermore, everyone who eats should read his book.

My "Concept of Totality" not only led to a lasting friendship with Dr. Fred Miller, it also brought me in touch with Dr. Henry Trautmann of Madison, Wisconsin. Both men were to be significant in the subsequent role I was to play in the natural food movement. Dr. Trautmann had suffered a coronary some time before and had moved from Brooklyn, where he had a hectic practice, to Wisconsin. He read my reprint and called me. He invited me to join him and a small group of physicians, dentists, and farmers in a meeting at the Normandy House Restaurant in Chicago. Similar small meetings had already been held. Dr. Trautmann assumed from what I had written in the "Concept" that I would be interested.

This was the beginning of NFA—Natural Food Associates. Whether it should be called its conception or its birth is difficult to determine. It is equally difficult to answer the question, Who started NFA?

My own association with this arm of the natural foods movement came after the preliminary steps had been taken toward organization. Apparently NFA started when Robert Rowe, who operated Hopewell Farms at Dalton City, Illinois, met Paul Pfund of Elenhurst, near Chicago, on January 6, 1952. As men of similar views, they soon developed a strong friendship. Pfund and two of his friends had already been discussing the need for an organization that would teach farmers how to restore and maintain the fertility of their soil. Rowe agreed, but felt an organization that also emphasized good food would have wider appeal.

Some of the early meetings were held at the home of Hamilton Noyes near Woodstock, Illinois. Those who attended these early meetings included Dr. Trautmann; Mrs. A. C. Leiter of Gurner, Illinois; Dr. Kenneth Ladwig of Naperville, Illinois; Dr. Royal Lee of Milwaukee, Wisconsin, and Ernest Halbleib, a very successful organic farmer from McNabb, Illinois. Halbleib took a very active part in the early meetings and on June 2, 1952, called a meeting at his farm. To this meeting he invited Dr. E. E. Pfeiffer and Peter Escher from Three Fold Farm in Spring Valley, New York. Dr. Pfeiffer's fame as a soil scientist had already spread around the world. At the time he was head of the Bio-Dynamic system of scientific farming.

With each meeting the movement gained impetus and its adherents nurtured enthusiasm. On October 12, 1952, Mr. and Mrs. Rowe hosted at their Hopewell Farms an organizational meeting for what was to become Natural Food Associates. Paul Pfund invited Alden Stahr of Starland Farm at Layton, New Jersey. Stahr was publisher and editor of *Normal Agriculture*, a four-page monthly publication devoted to natural farming methods and to nutrition. At this time Stahr offered to designate his periodical as the official publication of the new organization.

Robert Rowe served as chairman of a pro-tem committee for organization, assigned the duty of forming a permanent organization and selecting a board of directors. Other committeemen included Alden Stahr, vice chairman; Anthony Jackson of Assumption, Illinois, secretary-treasurer, and Dr. Trautmann, Mrs. Leiter, and Noyes. Rowe, who was responsible for the constitution and by-laws, obtained a charter from the State of Illinois for Natural Food Associates as a non-profit educational corporation. The charter bore the names of Rowe, Noyes, and Mrs. Leiter. The original board of directors included Gloria Swanson of New York City; Devin Garrity of New York City; Philip Wells of Haddon Heights, New Jersey; Mrs. Winslow S. Pierce of Dublin, New Hampshire; John Pearmain of Boston, Massachusetts; Lewis Eggleston of Davison, Michigan; Fred Engle of Muskegon, Michigan; L. P. DeWolf of Crescent City, Florida; E. H. Pratt of Kansas City, Missouri; Dr. Lee, Halbleib, and D. Earl Striplin of Tehachapi, California.

This was the state of NFA when I first became acquainted with it. The meeting to which Dr. Trautmann had invited me was the first annual directors meeting in Chicago on February 21-22, 1953. Both my education and my involvement grew rapidly from that point on.

When I checked into the headquarters hotel near the Normandy House Restaurant on the late afternoon of February 20, the lobby was empty. It was a 25-story hotel built before the turn of the century and my room cost only four dollars, but it had no bath. The bath was at the end of the hall. So I went back to the desk and for another dollar got a room with bath. Downstairs, nobody was in sight but the elevator boy and the desk clerk. I went into the drugstore. There I found the first proof that I had a fellow guest there. An old man, not so well dressed and lacking what I considered then to be the mark of an educated man, was buying a bottle of Mogen David wine.

I was lonesome and had to talk to somebody. I went up to the old man with my usual chamber of commerce approach.

"I'm Dr. Joe D. Nichols from Atlanta, Texas," I said as I stuck out my hand.

He was Dr. George Heard, a dentist from Hereford, Texas. He had come to Chicago to attend the NFA meeting. He paid for his wine and insisted that I join him in his room, which I was only too glad to do on that chilly, friendless Chicago afternoon.

In Dr. Heard's room that afternoon, I quickly realized I had an alert, educated, and knowledgeable man as my host. I was eager to hear his story and I soon learned that our histories were similar. He had lived in Tennessee, where he had become a victim of tuberculosis. He was told to go West for his health. He went to Hereford, out in the West Texas Panhandle country. Some of the most fertile soil in the world is in that part of Texas. The air was pure and the food was good—poison free and grown on fertile soil. He got well.

Hereford, Texas, was known as "The Town Without a Toothache." Some people ascribed the good dental health to the natural fluorine in the water. Dr. Heard was the only dentist there and he made very little money, but he did not go there to make money but to get well and he got well. Dr. Heard never agreed that the fluorine in Hereford's water accounted for the excellent dental health. He fought artificial fluoridation of the public water supplies as an unscientific hoax until his final breath. Since that day I met Dr. Heard, "scientific" farming methods have invaded Deaf Smith County, where Hereford is situated, and most of the people there today eat the "normal" American diet of overprocessed, devitalized, poisoned foods—and they have their share of toothaches, peridontal disease, and other common types of metabolic disease. Dr. Heard always insisted that natural food grown on fertile soil, not fluorine, had kept the toothaches away from Hereford.

By the time we had talked for several hours, I was hungry. I suggested he have dinner with me. But Dr. Heard offered an alternate plan. Why didn't I have dinner with him in his room?

It was a good thing Dr. Heard didn't feed me first, before telling his story. I would have thought him a "food nut." But by then he had given me a lecture on the evils of cooked foods, and I could see he looked healthy, even though he was an old man. So I was receptive, and I was hungry.

Dr. Heard had brought freshly-ground Deaf Smith County flour and some organically-grown Irish potatoes. With an old pocket knife he chopped up the potatoes and mixed them with the flour. Then he poured in a little wine and mixed it all together. Then he divided this concoction into the two bowls he had brought. The taste, to my surprise, was superb.

Years later I discovered that some of the world's best restaurants use raw potatoes and raw turnips as the basis for their most delicious salads.

The next morning at the Normandy House I met more odd and unusual people. Some of them looked sick. But so was I. Some of them held to what seemed to be "fanatical views." But so did I. However, some of them had solid knowledge about agriculture and nutrition, without a doubt. That was what I had come to Chicago to hear.

The first day we heard speeches. I gave a new speech I had developed on the occupational diseases of bankers, which William Philpott had urged me to write and which he had published in the *Texas Bankers Record.* And that night I listened to E. H. Pratt from Kansas City tell about his organic farm. He had, he explained, built up the fertility of the soil with compost, and he was producing a high-vitamin, high-mineral food supplement from the grasses grown on his farm. It sounded, frankly, a little quacky to me, but I listened, because I had a farm myself. By then I had learned a valuable lesson: not to discount what another man says just because it's new and different from what I'd been taught all my life. The man might have something valuable to give me, and the chances were it wouldn't cost me anything to find out. That night in Chicago, this was proved. My 1,000-acre farm, and I, benefitted immeasurably.

The next day we got down to business. We spent hours going over the proposed constitution. Bob Rowe and his associates had done a superb job.

Late that afternoon, a totally unexpected development materialized, one that was to change my life more than a little. Dr. Trautmann and Bob Rowe came to me. They asked me to become the national president of NFA. Why did they ask me? Well, I've always assumed it was because I was an M.D. and they knew I was chairman of the board of a bank and was from Texas. Texans, doctors, and bankers are all supposed to have money, and money was one thing NFA needed. They assumed I had money. I wasn't as well off as they probably assumed, but as one wag said, You don't have to have money, as long as everybody thinks you have! At first I demurred, but Dr. Trautmann was a very persuasive physician. On snap judgment, I accepted. It was one of the most fateful decisions I have ever made.

We adopted a seal at this meeting. The words *Natural Food Associates* proclaimed our organization across the top of the seal and on the bottom, *Better Foods From Living Soil.* Three sections of the seal displayed a green leaf for life and growth, a dead leaf for decay, and a compost pile for rebirth.

We were in business.

At our second annual meeting at the same Normandy House in Chicago, we agreed to produce our own magazine, to be called *Natural Food and Farming.* Robert Rowe was elected executive secretary and was to edit the publication. And I was reelected president. However, a week later, Robert Rowe called me. He had a 400-acre farm and a family that required his full time. Dr. Trautmann had persuaded him to accept the NFA role, but now he saw it was impossible. He insisted on resigning. By the time our telephone conversation was over, I had an additional burden of putting out a monthly magazine, along with being national president of NFA, not to mention the responsibilities of a busy medical practice.

I needed a solution fast. I searched my mind for a person I knew who could edit and publish *Natural Food and Farming.* Then I remembered Tom Lavin. Tom was my brother-in-law. He lived in Atlanta. As a musician and former band teacher, he had had experience in publishing a band camp magazine. So he knew how, and he was in Atlanta; if he would, we had it solved. At the time Tom was selling band instruments and uniforms to high schools over the Arkansas, Oklahoma, Texas and Louisiana region. When Tom got home one day I talked the proposal over with him. There was no money in the bank for a salary, but NFA needed a magazine and I needed an editor. Would he do it? After a while Tom agreed to put out the magazine if I would provide the material. And his wife, Julia—who was my sister—agreed to do the secretarial work for nothing. Our problem was solved and we were in business from that point on.

Volume I, Number 1 of *Natural Food and Farming* was published in April, 1954, and it has never missed a deadline since. I announced on the first "President's Page" that "We in Natural Food Associates have set out to change the eating habits of America." We felt the first issue made a good beginning. For it Dr. Royal Lee wrote an article on "The Special Nutritional Qualities of Natural Foods." Gloria Swanson contributed a column on "Glorious Living." The feature review was on that excellent book on ecology, *The Web of Life* by John H. Storer. The issue was a tangible confirmation of our existence.

As NFA grew, so did Tom Lavin's role. At first, NFA's national headquarters was in his living room. From the beginning he studied ways to improve and expand the magazine and soon he had sold enough advertising to pay for it. Whenever we could spare the time, Tom and I hit the road together, riding DC-3 airplanes at night to save money, going all over the country, telling the NFA story to whoever would listen. There soon were plenty of listeners. Everywhere we went, we met people who were ready and anxious to join NFA. Then ads for the magazine began to pour in. Some of them we couldn't accept—ads for magic potions, secret cures, and memberships in all kinds of lonely hearts clubs—for our advertising policy was as strict then as it is now (sometimes to the dismay of our advertising manager!). But most of the ads were legitimate and proved that our response was solid enough. We organized local chapters and state chapters all across the nation. NFA was on the way, and NFA was here to stay.

In reaching new minds, the purpose of NFA was, and is, two-fold:

1. To teach people the value of natural, poison-free food grown on fertile soil.

2. To help them get this food.

Deep within the collective psyche of NFA members was the belief that no man anywhere could ever violate any one of God's natural laws. The tenets that gave rise to NFA in the first place were the ones that nurtured us as we spoke to new groups and reemphasized our message to old friends. Briefly, the essential logic of NFA boiled down to these seven statements of belief:

1. America is a sick nation. Heart disease, cancer, diabetes, arthritis, dental caries, and many other metabolic diseases are rapidly increasing in this country. These are no longer diseases of old age. Our children are falling victim at an alarming rate.

2. The true prevention of these metabolic diseases can be found only in the practice of proper nutrition. Proper nutrition means natural food grown on fertile soil, eaten fresh and poison free. In the treatment of these diseases, proper nutrition is of paramount importance.

3. Although most Americans get enough calories, the quality of our food supply is woefully inadequate. Too many vitamins, minerals, enzymes, and essential fatty acids have been destroyed or lost in our modern processing and packaging of foods.

4. The fertility of our soils is rapidly declining, and our topsoil is being washed into the sea. Fertile soil is the greatest natural resource of any nation. Civilizations of the past have been destroyed when their fertile soils were lost.

5. Only a well-informed, aroused public can save America from poor food grown on poor soil. The addition of known cancer-causing chemicals to our food must be stopped.

6. Natural Food Associates is the one national organization that has the leadership, the courage, and the resources to bring these vital truths to our nation and to the world.

7. Everyone who eats should join Natural Food Associates.

We believe that modern "scientific" agricultural technology is an assault on nature, it is an ecological blunder, and that, left unchecked, it will destroy this nation and, perhaps, our planet. It has resulted in the universal pollution of our water, our soil, our food, and to some extent, our air. Modern food technology has resulted in our consuming overprocessed, devitalized food that contain dangerous chemical additives. This, plus modern agricultural technology, is directly responsible for the rapid increase of metabolic disease in this country. The present epidemic of cancer will never be slowed down or halted until our farmers and our food processors learn to respect natural laws. The present prevailing practices in agriculture and food technology are resulting in scientific suicide.

NFA was organized to work toward correcting these mistakes. So it was no surprise that, almost immediately after we had organized, the agricultural chemical industry and the food processors sought to discredit us. We were called food faddists, quacks, and charlatans. We were accused of that crime of crimes, of being unscientific. Our initial detractors were soon joined by the U.S. Department of Agriculture, the U.S. Department of Public Health through the Food and Drug Administration, and even the American Medical Association. A campaign was launched to make Americans believe our beliefs were myths. Newspaper and magazine articles, even entire books, were published in a gigantic effort to destroy the effect of NFA and our public credibility.

Attacking the food products that we considered harmful to Americans' health, we soon became personal targets of those who profited from selling these products to mass consumers. During a two-day seminar in Houston, Texas, I made the statement on radio that "The modern loaf of enriched white bread is not only worthless, but it's harmful. It is unfit for human consumption." Fearing, perhaps, that I might take white bread out of their customers' mouths, and money out of their pockets, the *Bakers Journal* responded with a full-page editorial calling me a quack and a food faddist, the old reliables of name-calling in the food processing industry.

About this time, in a seeming effort to discredit both our leaders and our objectives, the AMA and FDA Congress on Quackery went all over the United States, holding seminars on food faddism and quackery. Hospital dieticians, home economics teachers, and physicians were all invited. Some of the displays and demonstrations were certainly valid. They had examples of quack patent medicines and "miracle cures" and fantastic quack machines that were supposed to cure everything from lumbago to cancer. But you quickly got the impression all that was window-dressing. They were really after the men and women whose espousal of "natural foods" or "organic foods" or "health foods" threatened to lower the profits of the food industry.

I attended one of these seminars, without formal invitation, in McFarlin Auditorium at Southern Methodist University in Dallas. The star of the show was chairman of the Department of Nutrition at Harvard University's Medical School. He has insisted all along that all Americans need to do to get a perfectly healthy, nutritious diet is to go into any grocery store or supermarket and buy a variety of four basic food groups. On this occasion in Dallas, the professor became more personal. He incorporated into his remarks on food faddism and quackery the observation, "One of the biggest food faddists in the United States lives right here in Texas, and his name is Joe D. Nichols of Atlanta, Texas, the president of Natural Food Associates."

These were but some of the more obvious roadblocks thrown up in our early years. But the leaders of NFA have never let such attacks deter us from bringing the truth about proper nutrition to the American people. If anything, the attacks have increased our determination to tell our story. If our detractors insisted and persisted in going to such lengths to discredit us, it seemed to us, they had real doubts that the American people would continue to believe the White Bread, Sugar, and Hydrogenated Fat Story. Didn't they have deep anxieties about defending their products in the marketplace of ideas?

As early as 1953 we tried to tell America that DDT was a cancer-causing chemical. Our detractors pooh-poohed our words and called us quacks and faddists. Our charges against DDT were called a myth. Times have changed. The NFA story has proved itself to be true. Scientists all over America are now agreeing with the NFA story. All respectable scientists acknowledge DDT to be a cancer-causing chemical. The research to prove this was done by the Food and Drug Administration itself.

The attacks on us seem to be subsiding. They are subsiding because the food processors and the manufacturers of agricultural poisons are on the defensive. The people are beginning to learn the truth about their products. The ones who attacked us yesterday are on the run today. The tide is turning. And none too soon.

VI.

Human Ecology

I observe Earth Day every day, and every day is Earth Day for NFA. I am an ecologist. Everyone who belongs to Natural Food Associates is an ecologist. And we are but a few of the ecologists who are straining today to save this country and, in fact, the entire environment of this planet. For it is literally a question of all of us or none. The totality of the life on the total planet.

What is ecology?* It is the study of the interrelationships between organisms and their environments. I am convinced that conservation of soil, water, and human health are all interrelated. All living things—bacteria, insects, grass, birds, mammals—all fit into a pattern. The whole depends for its healthy existence upon the presence of each of its parts.

The *totality* of a person's adaptive responses is expressed by the term ecology, which was first used by Hoeckel in 1866 in referring to the mutual relations of organisms to their physical conditions of life, and to each other as described by Darwin. Human ecology embodies the concept of a person's adaptation to the conditions of his existence.

Ecology cannot be simplified. The universe is old and big

---

*I am indebted to my long-time friend and NFA colleague, Devin Garrity, for some of the ecological views given here, which he expressed in a speech, which impressed me.

and in motion. It has taken a long time to prepare a place on this earth for man to live. If we compare the earth to a 3,000-page book, with each page representing a million years, man would appear on the last page. Only the last two words would represent *civilized man*. Only the last dot would represent *scientific* man.

The earth is only a minute part of the limitless universe. To borrow another analogy, if we took a telescope and diligently and carefully studied outer space, we could only examine one square inch per year. How large and how old is the universe? These are questions so huge, so complex, so impossible to answer that they soon turn into philosophical and metaphysical discussions. But we do know that the universe, of which the earth is a microscopic part, is still in motion. There is a constant motion in all things, from the tiny atom to the circling of the earth around the sun. The negative electron in the atom circles the positive nucleus in an orderly manner. The earth itself is constantly turning on its axis. And all of this motion affects man and his environment. The moon, for example, controls the tides as well as exerting many other forces not well understood. And until scientific man came along and started tinkering with natural laws, things moved in harmony and in rhythm and in cycles.

The survival of man depends upon the survival of other life on this planet. In other words, he must fit in with his physical environment. His continued existence as a species depends on his obeying the natural laws written by the Creator, the slow accumulation of many millions of years. As a part of the whole picture, he is more sensitive to ecological change than many of the lesser animals and insects. Because man's generations are longer, he may be wiped out before he can adjust as a species. Man is not the be-all and end-all. He is but one part of the ecological mosaic. In one sense, it could be called an ecological house of cards: man shifts a card or two—and he falls too. He is, to a certain extent, a slave of his ecology. And the penalty for violating the laws of human ecology is death. And if man collectively violates these laws, then it means death to the species. Death has its own totality—and finality.

Chemical agriculture and the processed food industry are pulling down the ecological house of cards. If we continue, man will fall. Chemical agriculture and the anti-food industry, as it should be called, are destroying the ecological pattern developed over millions of years. They are doing it within the space of a generation. This comes as no news to anyone who has read any form of the printed word or has watched television over the past few years. It is common knowledge. Now it is an accepted fact that man must obey his ecological imperatives, or perish.

Our ecological decline is widespread. It almost staggers the mind to catalog the deterioration that is *known*.

Let us begin with the good earth. This is a good term. Without good, healthy earth we, the people who ultimately feed upon its products, will lose our health—as we are doing now, as multitudes of us have already done.

One of the little recognized threats to our country—and the world—today is that of soil erosion: the loss of humus and the leaching out of essential minerals from the soil. This is a greater threat than many of us realize, especially those of us in our modern urban civilization who are out of contact with the earth. But eight inches of topsoil, in which are found the earthworms, the soil bacteria, the fungi, and other, microscopic forms of life, provide the true means of support for all life on this planet: vegetation, trees, insects, animals, human beings.

Without proper care, good healthy topsoil can, over a period of time, wash and blow away, leaving behind a desert. Grasses, shrubs, and trees help keep the soil from eroding. Dead leaves and decaying vegetation not only add nutrients to the soil, they hold water and at the same time protect from heavy, washing rains. Over and over again, forests are being destroyed by fire and overcutting. Overgrazing keeps the grass and shrubs down. Unwise cultivation practices add to the burden. The hot sunshine burns up oxidized humus. As a result of all these usually man-related activities, an accelerated kind of erosion has been occurring for the past 250 years, doing more soil damage over the world than in all the time before then.

We might refer to this as the "erosion explosion," for that is just what it is; in the long run, it may be the most serious "explosion" we shall have to face.

It is a world-wide tragedy: both North and South America, all of West Asia, China, Australia, India, Africa, most of the countries around the Mediterranean. One-third of our country's arable topsoil has washed into the sea over the years, and it is still being lost faster than we can conserve it. Since the Pilgrims came to America, we have probably stripped nine-tenths of our forest lands, and each year we are still cutting more than we replace. As far as the soil is concerned, we have probably wasted as much as half of our continent's fertility. At the rate we are going, we can expect to have lost three-fourths of our fertile soil by the end of this century—now less than three decades off. Soil erosion costs us 500,000 acres of good land each year. During the Missouri River basin floods of July, 1947, for example, more than 115 million *tons* of rich topsoil were washed downstream by the rains.

Only in Europe have conservation efforts been able to keep up with erosion. Dam building doesn't provide the answer; reservoirs tend to fill up with silt in about thirty-five years, as has happened to hundreds of reservoirs in the United States. In a sediment survey made in Japan in 1950, twenty-four of fifty-four artificial reservoirs were more than half-filled with sediment. In a mere eighteen years those twenty-four reservoirs had lost an average of 73 per cent of their water storage capacity!

These facts point out one thing forcibly, that prevention is dramatically more effective than repair.

The destruction endured by our woodlands in recent years is a vital part of the "erosion explosion." In time the loss of trees contributes to the erosion of the soil. Along with fires, the industrial users of timber and paper pulp take a frightening toll of forests. Wood consumption in Europe exceeds new forest growth by from 10 to 15 per cent. The excess in this country is even greater. One example will help to fix the picture in one's mind. A single edition of the Sunday *New York Times* used enough wood pulp to chew up 10 acres of big trees. A high figure? Yes, but it is a conservative one. Estimates have gone as high as *100* acres.

Perhaps many will not see the urgent connection between soil erosion and other issues closer to home for most of us. The fact is, though, that soil erosion plays a large role in our growing crisis related to a diminished supply of high quality food. Tied to the reality of a booming world population that has proliferated over the past 250 years, high quality food becomes even more precious. We have reached a hitherto unheard-of state of affairs: there are more people than can be adequately fed from the existing fertile soil. Individual, governmental, and United Nations authorities agree on this.

What are we to do? How must we approach this world-wide crisis? W. C. Lowdermilk, in a U.S. Soil Conservation Service publication, *Conquest of the Land Through 7,000 Years,** saw the need for a swift change of heart, when he wrote: "If civilization is to avoid a long decline such as has blighted North Africa and the Near East for thirteen centuries and for centuries yet to come, society must be born again out of an economy of exploitation into an economy of conservation." In other words, we must work with nature, as a friend, instead of exploiting her, as an enemy.

The facts are simple. Population is increasing. Good land on which we can grow quality food is decreasing. And mere application of NKP fertilizer is not going to solve our problem.

I have seen several aspects of this world-wide problem in my own backyard. During World War II, my home county in East Texas had fifty-seven "peckerwood" sawmills in addition to the larger mills. A peckerwood sawmill might be called a fly-by-night operation; it is a small operation that sets up in a woods and saws away until the timber is stripped; it riddles the woods like a peckerwood works over a dead tree. Ecology is served by the peckerwood's activities, but not by the peckerwood sawmill. These mills cut everything that would make a two-by-four.

The open fields were cultivated to death. Everyone seemed to concentrate on meeting the needs of the war effort, with more food and fiber for more money. This great push for quantity production was carried out with little, if any, thought of conservation of the natural resources. The war, consequently, almost ruined our lands and our economy. Our springs dried up in the summertime. We had a terrible drouth. The heavy spring rains could not penetrate into the soils; our precious topsoil was washed into the Gulf of Mexico.

One-fourth of our population—10,000 persons—left our rural areas because they could no longer eke out a living on their farms and ranches. The land would not grow cotton and corn any longer. One after another, the sawmills and the cotton gins closed. In town, the merchants saw their business volume sag. The young people began to move elsewhere, making their homes where they could find opportunity. In my hospital, the obstetrical department got less and less busy. And there were other symptoms or warnings. New fauna began to appear. Roadrunners, rattlesnakes, and

----

*USDA Information Bulletin #99 (August, 1953).

armadillos moved in. In more ways than one, the desert was moving our way.

In this moment of crisis, a new organization stepped in to fight the battle, to at least ward off the desert's encroachment. The Marion-Cass Soil Conservation District called a meeting of civic leaders and U.S. Department of Agriculture personnel in the area. I was proud to be a member of that district, and I still am.

We made a survey. We learned that we had 250,000 acres that needed to be planted in winter cover crops. Vetch, crimson clover, Austrian winter grass, oats, and rye—these would both protect the land from further erosion and restore the fertility of the soil.

We were determined to save our soil and water. We forgot about terraces and mechanical conservation measures. We set out to plant pine trees and winter cover crops. One year we planted 10 *million* pine seedlings. We began turning the district green with grass and winter legumes that would put natural nitrogen back into the soil. Our springs began coming back to life. Good cattle soon dotted the pastures that once would not support "scrub" cows.

All this was accomplished through use of local funding—an auction sale of rusted machinery, loans from now-interested bankers—but we didn't hesitate to call upon various governmental agencies for other forms of help. Soil Conservation Service technicians, the Texas Forest Service, vocational agriculture teachers, home demonstration agents all joined to help at our regular monthly meetings.

At one time, when there was a large rural population, there were no roads. Then, later remedying this, farm-to-market state highways were built all over the district. But by this time hardly anybody lived there any more. Today, however, the roads are highly practical, for new brick homes are being built on these once-forsaken roads.

A dead county, or area, can come back to life. Ours has done it. In fact, in the mid-1950s our district won the prize as the district making the best use of all agencies, and in 1957 and 1958 we won the Goodyear Award for our conservation efforts.

At the same time, it is only a beginning and perhaps it is a sad commentary on the condition of our land in this country that our district won these awards. We still have many acres to put in pines and winter cover crops. When we accepted our first prize I said, "If we won it, God pity the rest of you!" I didn't think we had done anything worth bragging about.

But the enemies of proper soil conservation and human ecology continue, even in my own county where, as I said, we have made progress. Although there are hopeful signs that our nation is waking up to its ecological crisis, there is also proof that the same old approach that brought us to this crisis is still the dominant one in this country. I refer to "modern scientific methods" of agriculture.

As for quantity, there is no argument that these methods bring almost immediate results. It is possible to produce three bales of cotton where only one grew before. Thanks to modern chemical fertilizers and pesticides, three blades of grass grow where only one grew before. Scientific agricultural practices have enabled the American farmer to produce a vast surplus of food for our people.

At the turn of the century, it took one man to produce enough food for three others. Today, one man can produce enough for forty other persons. Progress has been so great in producing quantity that the government now pays farmers to keep portions of their land idle. We have built thousands of new warehouses to store surplus grains.

Yet these agricultural accomplishments are only a part of what "science" has brought us in late twentieth-century America. Let us look a little further.

Modern science and technology have brought to the American housewife an almost unlimited supply of foods from all over the world. The keeping qualities of these foods are such that they do not even need refrigeration. How is this? Well, the addition of chemicals will prevent spoilage for weeks. Furthermore, chemical additives make modern foods look fresh, soft, and tempting. Our modern bakeries produce a loaf of bread that is soft and smooth. It stays fresh for days. Food technologists have designed TV dinners that are easy to prepare. Just heat and eat, as it says in the ad. Even inexperienced bachelors can prepare dinner in a few minutes with these pre-cooked foods.

Nor are big city supermarket shoppers the only beneficiaries of these scientific "advances." A wide variety of pre-cooked cereals, many of which are already sugar-coated, can be found in almost any country grocery store in the most isolated area. The food processing industry has saturated every nook and cranny of our country with its products.

Worm-free, beautifully colored fruit and exotic foods from around the world are readily available in all America. Modern containers and packages, sometimes containing insect repellents, make them "safe" and "pure" and resistant to spoilage. Citrus fruits can be harvested in a pre-ripened state that gives them keeping qualities unheard of in the old days. Green-wrapped tomatoes harvested in June are available in the winter months all over the nation.

And this is but the beginning. Vitamin-deficient breads and cereals that once produced beriberi and other vitamin B-deficiency diseases are no longer a problem. These breads and cereals are now enriched with the precious B vitamins. Foods are also enriched with vitamins A and D, which is said to control night blindness and rickets. Beautiful, artificially-colored and flavored "orange" drinks now contain more vitamin C than natural orange juice—and cost less. In fact, modern technology has produced these chemical vitamin additives so cheaply that these enriched foods cost even less than the foods that contain these nutrients naturally.

It is even more amazing what American know-how has done when we stop to realize that technology has milled the food substances, thereby removing some of the vitamins and minerals, and then has gone back and restored several of them—and the whole process is done so cheaply that the resulting food costs less than it would cost without it. At least, this is what we are told.

There seems to be no limit to what wonderful products science can bring us. Now there are ways to irradiate foods to prevent spoilage. Bacon can be irradiated and kept for years. Irish potatoes can be irradiated to prevent sprouting. Irradiated steaks have keeping qualities never before heard of.

Modern insecticides have come to our rescue. Malaria, encephalitis, yellow fever, and typhus, all of which once raged in epidemics, are almost under control. The modern, postwar chlorinated hydrocarbon and phosphorus compounds promise to eradicate the vectors that transmit these diseases. DDT, the granddaddy of them all, is cheap and is easily applied with modern spray machines. The modern airplane has been easily adapted to spread them on vast marshlands and other hard-to-reach areas.

The deadly fire ant, which once threatened areas of the

Southern states, has been partially controlled by mass spraying of insecticides. Mass sprayings with deadly insecticides is a product of modern science and technology.

And now, from those wonderful people who gave us DDT and white enriched bread and chemical additives and white sugar and sodium cyclamates, we learn that America is a healthy nation and that our food supply is safe, abundant, and nourishing.

We never had it so good. We have come into a paradise on earth. Is that not the message we have been told, time after time?

Those of us who may have accepted that message must have been stunned when we heard, as long ago as 1964, President Lyndon B. Johnson's health message to the Congress.

"Cancer, heart disease, and strokes stubbornly remain the leading causes of death in the United States," said President Johnson. "They now afflict fifteen million Americans—two-thirds of all Americans now living will ultimately suffer or die from one of them.

"These diseases are not confined to older people. Approximately half of the cases of cancer are found among persons under sixty-five. Cancer causes more deaths among children under age fifteen than any other disease.

"More than half the persons suffering from heart disease are in their most productive years. Fully a third of all persons with recent strokes or with paralysis due to strokes are under sixty-five."

When the President of the United States himself acknowledges these unsavory facts, we are faced with the inescapable conclusion that America is *not* a healthy nation. Surely this Presidential confirmation must have come as shocking news to some of the biochemists who have traveled across the nation lecturing us on how healthy science and industry had made us. But it was old news to most Americans. They had already seen sickness in their families or friends, or had experienced it themselves.

This is the reason Americans have become frantic in their search for health. In recent years they have submitted their own bodies and the bodies of their loved ones to all kinds of miracle cures and quackery. And cancer, heart disease, and stroke have continued to take their deadly tolls, despite the skills and false promises of both the scientific community and other less respected healers.

Despite the three billions that the President's commission

recommended as needed to combat these dread diseases, and the national network of diagnostic and treatment stations, I was unable to find anywhere any request for methods to really prevent the basic cause of these diseases. It did ask for $10 million for a comprehensive national program of education regarding the hazards of cigarette smoking. But nowhere in the report did I find any mention of the dangers of modern insecticides, food additives, and processed foods. Surgery, cobalt machines, and mechanical devices were the chief weapons asked for to halt the death rate from cancer, heart disease, and stroke.

Their recommendations will not prevent heart disease, cancer, and stroke. Modern science and technology have failed. Despite all the progress we mentioned earlier, our society now has more sickness, more unhappiness and frustration. Are these harmful side effects necessary? Must technological progress in agriculture be accompanied by mass poisoning of our food, our air, and our water? Must progress in food technology be accompanied by a host of overprocessed, devitalized empty calories that lead to obesity, dental caries, and a long list of other metabolic diseases?

Who is responsible for our present failure of technology? Who is responsible for the devastating side effects of mass spraying with modern insecticides? Who is responsible for the harmful effects of many of the food additives? Who is responsible for the nitrate poisoning caused by the excessive use of synthetic nitrogen on our farms? Who is responsible for the pollution of our waters with detergents?

I say they are responsible who have actively supported and worked to establish and maintain these dangerous teehnological errors in our civilizaztion, even if it was merely by endorsement. I agree with Dr. Aaron J. Ihde, professor of chemistry at the University of Wisconsin, who said, "The scientist seeking to apply a new development has a responsibility to anticipate overall effects, not merely the favorable effects." There are some scientists, Dr. Ihde continued, who claim "it is not possible for the investigator to foresee the use which will be made of his discoveries, therefore his only responsibility is to discover. I take issue with this position, feeling that scientists are also members of the human race and have a responsibility for the preservation and extension of civilization."

I cannot overemphasize my own agreement with Dr. Ihde's words. One of the best illustrations of the form of scientist he was speaking of is seen in the program that was undertaken to eradicate the Aedes Aegypti mosquito in ten Southern states. This mosquito is the vector of yellow fever. Although there had not been a recorded case of yellow fever in America in more than 50 years, millions of dollars were spent by the government to mass-spray the area in a vain attempt to eradicate the mosquito. Similar attempts to eradicate insects by mass spraying have always failed, and the damage done to fish and wildlife and to man is now well known. Yet the U.S. Public Health Service, the Pan American Health Organization, and other scientific organizations endorsed the program. Unfortunately, the endorsements did nothing to prevent the damage done by the mass spraying. What may be even more unfortunate, endorsements by scientific organizations and governmental agencies can no longer be depended upon to insure safety.

Applied science has, too often, come to mean a study directed toward a definite objective regardless of the side effects. The objective I am speaking of is *money*. The expected profit in much of today's research is the guiding motivation, and this motive often blinds the researcher to the possibility of harmful effects. In recent years, it has even been alleged that, in many instances at least, the recipient of a research grant is required to give the grantor a confidential report. Then the grantor decides whether or not the experiment results are made public. His decision, of course, is dictated by the knowledge that such publicity will help or hurt his company. Money again rules. Both industry and government supply enormous sums of money for this type of research. The system is so firmly established in our country, and so permeating, that it is no easy task to decide where, exactly, reform must begin.

In agriculture most of the research is an effort to make more bushels per acre at less cost. Farmers are taught at our best universities that for every dollar they spend on plant foods (*i.e.*, synthetic nitrogen, inorganic salts, NKP—what was formerly referred to as commercial fertilizer), they can expect a return of three or four extra dollars. Most of the farmers believed these "authoritative" statements, for sales are at an all-time high. But after years of continued use, the farmer found that nematodes and insects have become a problem of escalating significance. Disease in his plants is now quite common.

The chemical industry replied with more research, more

scientific answers. Chemistry was the answer. A new term even appeared: chemurgy. Chemurgy was the application of science to agriculture. It became big business.

By 1975, it has been estimated by the National Chemicals Association, $1 billion will be spent for agricultural chemicals. Yet the farm problem grows worse annually, and thousands of farmers leave the land each year.

This is the kind of science that will destroy us.

There are some areas in which it should be obvious, even to the most unsophisticated mind, that extreme care should be taken to protect the consumer. One of these is any process that is undertaken strictly to extend the shelf life of a commercial product. This should especially be true of irradiation, such as I have spoken of. The NFA policy is, *Never eat a food that won't spoil, but eat it before it does.* We do not know exactly what irradiation does, but the safety has not been proved. Nor do we believe the safety of the microwave oven has been proved. In my opinion, it would take generations to prove irradiation of foodstuffs is safe—if it can be proved.

A true scientist should not be obligated to anything except a search for truth. We need more research by honest scientists who are interested in "pure science," an attempt to find truths related to natural law.

Science, many have suggested, has become the handmaiden of industry. Continued grants for research depend sometimes on a conformity to the predetermined wishes of the grantor. Too often this stifles independent thinking and honest research; sometimes the researcher is unaware of the limitations the grant has put upon him. For example, continued grants for research in food technology usually depend on producing a product that has shelf life and that is attractive enough to be sold in the supermarket for a profit by a food processor and grant giver.

For years this country has allowed residues of poisonous sprays on our food. This is another instance of misapplied science. Rachel Carson, both a distinguished and courageous scientist herself, documented the threat of these pesticides in her mind-awakening *Silent Spring*. The book became a best-seller. Justice William O. Douglas called it "the most important chronicle of this century for the human race." But some scientists immediately attacked Miss Carson's work. They attacked her vehemently. What would you expect from the National Manufacturers Chemical Association and the scientists who do research sponsored by them? Miss Carson had probed in their most sensitive nerve, the one stretching from the area of their pocketbook. They were not free to view her work objectively.

Miss Carson quoted Dr. William C. Hueper of the National Cancer Institute, a foremost authority on environmental cancer, as saying that DDT is a chemical carcinogen. Yet it has been practically impossible to go into the modern supermarket and buy fruits and vegetables untouched by this cancer-causing poison. The Food and Drug Administration set a tolerance of no more than 7 parts per million for DDT. But no more than six-tenths of 1 per cent of the fruits and vegetables have been examined. There are not enough inspectors. Thus, not only has it become legal to expose the general population to a highly poisonous, cancer-causing pesticide, there is no way to regulate strictly its use on our food. How many of the foodstuffs that *weren't* inspected contained more than 7 parts of DDT per million? At least today we have seen some action taken on DDT, but it has not been aggressive enough, nor effective. The same is true of many, many other dangerous pesticides.

Since 1950, reported Miss Carson, deaths from all types of malignancies of the blood and the lymph increased sharply. Dr. Malcolm Hargraves and associates in the hematology department at the Mayo Clinic stated that "almost without exception these patients have a history of exposure to various toxic chemicals, including sprays which contains DDT, chlordane, benzene, lindane, and petroleum distillates."

In 1963 Dr. Hueper was quoted in the *Medical World News* as saying that "man-made environmental carcinogens have created, and continue to create, a serious threat to human health and life." Dr. Hueper's 47-page report to the New York Academy of Sciences noted that "once an epidemic of cancer from such sources has been started, there are at present no effective means available to arrest or modify its course for the individuals who have effectively become exposed to the carcinogenic agent."

Dr. Hueper pointed out that during the past century man has become exposed to increasing cancer hazards as a result of four factors: the increase in amounts of man-made carcinogens; an increase in the contact made by man to these chemicals; an increase in the spread of these chemicals into the general environment of plants and animals, and an increase in the resistance of "economically interested parties responsible for these hazards" to enforcement of control measures.

We continue to hear voices saying that our exploding population cannot be fed without the use of these poisons. To me this is ridiculous. We fed our people before World War II without these wide-spectrum pesticides. We can do it again. But to do so we must follow the advice of those scientists who know that we can grow not only quality, but quantity too, with natural organic farming methods. It is being done on thousands of American farms today.

It has been charged that abandonment of these known cancer-causing chemicals would create chaos in the chemical industry. This may be so. But which is worse, chaos in the chemical industry or chaos in the health of all our people? I am convinced we must return to sane practices that will insure the people's health, if we are to survive as a nation.

Certainly this is not going to be an easy task, to change the course of this nation—and perhaps this globe—from one of misapplied science to responsible ecology. It is a waste of time to condemn any individual scientist or organization. When we look closely at the way things are going today, it is difficult to blame or condemn the soil scientist very much. He has been taught in the modern university to believe he is doing good for humanity. He has observed, and perhaps participated in, what is now called applied science.

We would be better off and more effective if we took aim at the system that nurtures these practices. Controlled grants for research make it almost impossible to teach modern organic farming methods in a state university. This must be changed. The dismal failure of this system, in time, would spell its own doom, but it would bring your doom and my doom along with it. We can't afford to sit idly by and wait for the system to fail. Most of us have children or grandchildren. We can't wait for this materialistic system to destroy our generations while proving itself invalid.

The sober ecologist must replace the drunken driver of modern science.

VII.

Meanwhile, Down at the Cell

When I studied histology in medical school, about all I saw in the human cell under the microscope was the nucleus, which contained a little shadow, and a blob of "empty jelly." Today with the new powerful electron microscope we can see the anatomy of the cell. Within the nucleus we can see the "blueprint," which is called the DNA, deoxyribonucleic acid. The shadow in the nucleus is the RNA, ribonucleic acid, the messenger. And now in what was formerly called empty jelly, we can see the centrosomes and the Golgi bodies, which have been called the packaging plant. We can see the long worm-like structure, the endoplasmic reticulum. And on these you can see the ribosomes. The mitochondria are bean-shaped bodies. These are the organelles which have to do with a process called metabolism.

The food that we eat is digested and absorbed from the intestine into the blood stream. Essential nutrients are carried to the individual cells all over the body. All our energy, growth, and repair come from these individual cells through this process of metabolism. It is amazing what the capacity is for this cell to repair itself *provided* it gets proper nutrition.

We have made great progress in the prevention of infectious diseases, both bacterial and viral. But we have made practically no progress in the prevention of metabolic disease, and we will

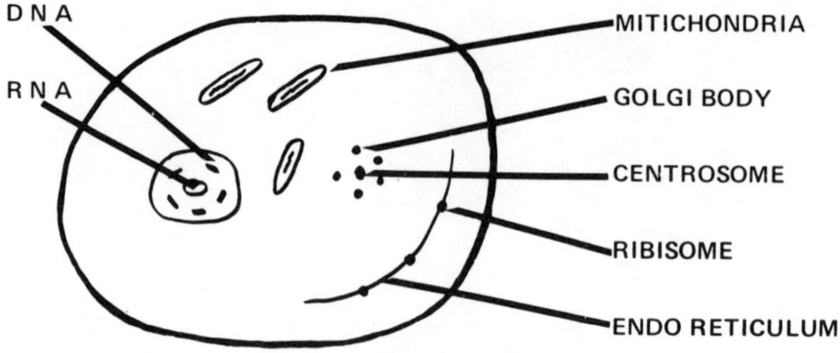

THE HUMAN CELL

never prevent metabolic disease until we learn how to give our people proper nutrition.

What is proper nutrition? I agree with Dr. Roger Williams of the University of Texas: *Proper nutrition is like a chain. If any single link is missing, some type of metabolic disease will result.* This is the importance of the cell. Life begins, and ends, at the cell. The cell is the basic unit of life. It is where the action is. Metabolism occurs in the cell, and this is why a good nutritionist must be interested in what goes into that cell.

Dr. Seymour Lionel Halpern, one of our great authorities on nutrition, has said that in order to get proper nutrition one must have all the essential nutrients, simultaneously, and in balance.*

This means that we must have all the essential amino acids, as well as other factors.

	1. 8 Essential Amino Acids
All	2. Natural Vitamins
–	3. Organic Minerals
Simultaneously	4. 3 Essential Fatty Acids
–	5. Unrefined Carbohydrates
In Balance	6. Unknown factors.

How do you get all the essential nutrients simultaneously and in balance? That is where the argument starts. There are some who say that all one has to do is get a wide variety of the four great food groups. These are: bread and cereals, fruits and vegetables, meat and eggs, and dairy products. They say these can be found in any modern supermarket. Their claim is not true. It is almost impossible to get proper nutrition at the modern

**Annals, New York Academy of Science* (1958:63), p. 147.

supermarket. Most Americans do not know how to read a label, and even if they did it would be almost impossible to find good natural, poison-free food in the supermarket.

Another group of enthusiasts have come to believe that they can continue eating junk foods and still get proper nutrition by taking added vitamins and mineral supplements. I cannot agree with them.

I do not believe one can continue to eat refined salt, hydrogenated fats, white flour, sugar, glucose, and the refined cereals and escape metabolic disease.

The real answer to proper nutrition is food, not pills. The real answer is natural, poison-free food grown on fertile soil, eaten fresh, and not overcooked. This is the way to get all the essential nutrients in balance.

I am well aware that there is not enough of this type food in America today to feed the country. But the supply is increasing. Only an increased demand will bring an increased supply. Until you can get these foods you will need to take extra supplements. But you can get an education and you can learn how to avoid junk foods. This is the purpose of this book.

Many people have deficiencies of specific nutrients and require specific vitamins and mineral supplements. I think all cardiovascular patients should have additional vitamin E. This includes all diabetics. Certain types of rheumatism benefit from additional vitamin B_6. The patient who has bleeding gums and bruises easily requires additional natural vitamin C until the condition has been corrected. These are just examples. Scores of other metabolic diseases can be helped by additional supplements.

Proper nutrition is not easy to get in America today. The purpose of Natural Food Associates is to show the people everywhere how and where to get proper nutrition. An education is the first requirement. That is why we have three printing presses on which we produce a monthly magazine, a newspaper, and millions of reprints. That is why we travel all over the country holding two-day seminars wherever we can get people to come and listen to the NFA story.

If you cannot get proper nutrition in the modern supermarket, where can you get it? The health food store does not have all of it, but most of these have the whole grains, oils, peanut butter, poison-free fruits, and many other products that are acceptable. Recently their numbers are increasing, and many now have poison-free vegetables. Thousands of city dwellers now have organic backyard gardens where they grow their own poison-free vegetables. This book will show you how to grow a backyard garden.

This is the NFA story, then: if you put proper nutrition into that cell without poisons, then the cell has an amazing ability to regenerate itself. It can repair itself. But for proper nutrition, you must have *all* the essential nutrients. Proper nutrition, let us remember, is a *chain*, not a raggedy rope that has to be reinforced with supplementary strings here and there. Every single link of the chain must be present.

The word *essential* means exactly what it says. You *must* have all eight of the essential amino acids that compose our protein structures. The amino acids are our building blocks. If even one is absent, then we have a missing link in our chain of life.

Furthermore, there are five other nutrients that are essential to good health, besides the amino acids. We must also have natural vitamins, organic minerals, the essential fatty acids, unrefined carbohydrates, and the *essential unknown factors*.

You have not heard much about the essential unknown factors, so I will take this up first. I cannot tell you what the unknown factors are, of course, but I am not afraid to admit that they do exist. Otherwise, I would be saying that I know every last microscopic ingredient in every item of food—a grossly egotistical statement, I am sure you would say. Yet when we fail to acknowledge the unknown factors in food, we are claiming such all-knowledge—and basing it on the partial knowledge that we have already learned in the laboratories.

One of our most respected biochemists once made the statement that cobalt was not necessary to human nutrition. A few months later vitamin B_{12} was discovered. Vitamin B_{12} contains cobalt. Cobalt *is* an essential nutrient. Previously unknown factors are being discovered continually, and I suspect this pattern will continue as long as man is here. Just relatively recently, researchers found a factor in natural safflower oil that prevented muscular dystrophy in mice. It was an essential unknown factor.

Recently a newly discovered group of substances obtained from certain natural foods was shown to prevent typhoid infection in mice and chickens. This has given us the basis for a postulate of a new defense strategy against disease. Dr. Howard A. Schneider, formerly director of the Laboratory of Experimental Ecology at the Rockefeller Institute and later with the A.M.A. Institute for Biomedical Research, has called these compounds "pacifarins" because of their ability to pacify disease organisms. They were previously unknown compounds. Working with mice and mouse typhoid caused by Salmonella, utilizing pacifarin extracted from wheat and dried egg white, Dr. Schneider said, "Researchers may not only be able to explain non-genetic aspects of natural resistance, but they possibly could provide such resistance *dietarily.*"

Dr. Schneider went on to explain that "the collision of a disease organism with a susceptible individual does not automatically result in disease. What has been made increasingly clear in these affairs is that, although the pathogen is a necessary condition for disease, it is not a sufficient condition. Before disease can occur there must be an interaction between pathogen and host. The presence of a pacifarin seems to muffle this interaction. Host and pathogen settle down to a harmless association."

Dr. Schneider explained that the pacifarin does not destroy bacteria. Nor does it trigger an immune mechanism. It is not a vitamin or a mineral, but it is found in foods. I believe Sir Albert Howard was suggesting the same thing decades ago when he demonstrated that cattle grazed on fertile soils possessed some sort of unknown resistance to hoof and mouth disease. Could it be that pacifarins are more abundant in foods grown on fertile soils?

The unknown factors have always been found in the same place—natural food. This is because nature has put them there in the first place. After all, our synthetic vitamins and minerals are made in laboratories, but they necessarily are copies from nature's models. If we do not know the model—and how can we when the factor is unknown?—then there is no way any researcher in any laboratory can copy it.

This, once admitted, must surely be a frustrating piece of knowledge to a refined food faddist.

Now let us return to the *natural* vitamins that are essential to proper nutrition and good health. You must have all of the natural vitamins. Everyone, I think, accepts the argument that you must have all the essential vitamins, but here again the arguments vary. Some say synthetic vitamins are just as good and that there is no difference between laboratory-synthesized vitamins and the natural ones found in food. But there is a difference. Biochemists may disagree with me here, and up to a point they are right. There is no *chemical* difference. But there is a *biological* difference, and this is extremely important.

Let us take vitamin B_1 for an illustration. If you put synthetic vitamin B_1 before the polariscope—an instrument for looking at things in polarized light—you find that it has no motion. It is racemic, or motionless. On the other hand, if you put natural vitamin B_1 before the polariscope, it rotates to the right. It is dextrorotary. Therefore, there is a physical difference between natural and synthetic vitamins. Nature seems to have a right-handed twist.

There is another difference. Natural vitamins are never found in pure crystalline states. They are always found in association with other parts of a complex and also in combination with other vitamins and/or minerals. This is a biological difference and should be taken into consideration in weighing the relative values of natural and synthetic vitamins.

Our essential minerals also should be organic. Inorganic minerals are toxic and in sufficient quantity this is demonstrated. A leading cause of death in small children is iron intoxication, or poisoning. It comes from inorganic iron supplements. The baby gets Mama's bottle of iron pills. The baby eats too many. It kills the baby. Organic minerals are found in natural food. Organic minerals, like vitamins, are in balanced proportions in natural food. Turnip greens, grown on fertile soil, have lots of healthful, blood-enriching iron in them. So do other foods grown on fertile soil that has iron in it to begin with.

I have said that we must have all the essential nutrients. We also must have them simultaneously. In other words, if you get four amino acids for breakfast and four for supper, that won't do. You would be like the eight-cylinder automobile hitting on four; that automobile is sick. You need all eight of the essential amino acids for breakfast, as well as for the other two meals each day. A man who eats a piece of white bread toasted and coated with margarine, which you might call a synthetic butter, and washes it down with a cup of coffee does not get all eight amino acids. And that glazed doughnut he eats later on in the morning doesn't help him any either; in fact, he's worse off eating than not.

I have stated we need *all* the essential nutrients, we need them *simultaneously*, and now, thirdly, we need them in *balance*. Balance, I am convinced, is the secret, not only of good nutrition and health, but of life itself.

But this sounds terribly complicated, you may say! All the essential nutrients, as I have described them, simultaneously, and in balance. Doesn't this mean we must pedantically examine every morsel that goes into our mouths, practically weigh it as must the calorie-counters who have been placed on special gram-conscious diets?

Not at all. Nothing could be farther from the truth. Relatively speaking, our task is simple. We have working for us here the fact that natural food is automatically in balance. It just grows that way. Its composition derives from nature's millions of years. As long as we consume a variety of natural foods, we are assured of their balanced nutritional value that gives us a simultaneous nutritional feast. If we see that we get all the essential nutrients from natural foods, the rest happens automatically. You might even say it comes naturally.

Then how do you get it?

I make two lists. One is negative, one positive. One tells you what to avoid. The other tells you what to use. There are five food items the patient must avoid if he is to take the first steps toward healthful eating. Although this seems negative, since it is basically avoidance, it is also positive, for what it amounts to is the avoidance of negative factors in the diet. These five are:

1. *Refined* salt.
2. Hydrogenated fats.
3. White flour.
4. White sugar and glucose.
5. Most dry cereals.

By simply avoiding these, you automatically improve your health. These are the five most negative factors in the American diet today. I would not hesitate to call them "nutrition pollutants" in our ecology-conscious society today. They are harmful. When harmful items are removed from the diet, the consumer *has* to benefit, just as one improves, certainly, when poisons are eliminated from his food or atmosphere.

Let us begin with our first item, refined salt. Refined table salt, or sodium chloride, is toxic. It is not as toxic in small quantities as are certain other substances listed in the Merck Index of Toxicology, but it is bad enough to cause high blood pressure and heart disease, as has been demonstrated in the medical literature. Refined salt is different from other, natural salt in that all the trace minerals found with it have been taken out. When it reaches the supermarket and, from there, the table, it is pure sodium chloride. Nor is this all. This is further treated under high heat with sodium silicate, a drying agent, which makes it free-flowing in wet weather. Unfortunately, this disturbs the balance of sodium and potassium at the cellular level of the heart. This means, eventually, heart disease. We have spoken of autopsies that showed three-year-olds to have had lesions in the aorta of the heart. One of the reasons, beyond a doubt, is that commercial baby food contained refined salt. Ironically, this was placed in baby food strictly to please Mama who tasted the mushy contents of the little jars before feeding them to Junior. The baby couldn't have cared less whether it was salty or not. And if the mother had known what she was doing to Junior's heart, she undoubtedly would have cared more.

Hydrogenated fats, number two on our list, is the Number One cause of heart disease today, in my opinion. By hydrogenated fats I mean the fats and oils that commonly are found in shortening, mellorine, most store-bought peanut butter, practically all the commercial bakery products, crackers, cookies, and breads—including most of the whole grain breads in our great supermarkets. Mellorine, sold widely in the South, is a cheap substitute for ice cream that has been made from hydrogenated oils.

Okay, Doctor, you may say, but what makes hydrogenated fats so wrong and dangerous? How's it so different from natural fats and oils?

This: Linolenic acid has eighteen carbon atoms. Of those eighteen carbon atoms, there are four spots where there is no hydrogen. This means that, in time, it will spoil and become rancid. We can depict it like this:

```
                       H H   H H
     H H H H H H H H H     H     H H H H
H--- C C C C C C C C C C C C C C C C C C ---H
     H H H H H H H H H H H H H H H H H H
```

NICKEL

HEAT

Thus, in the natural state linolenic acid is a polyunsaturate. You can see the four spots in which there is no hydrogen.

But the food processor wasn't content to continue dealing with a product that would eventually spoil if left on the shelf. He began experimenting. He discovered that if he added nickel for a catalyst, and heated it, he could force hydrogen into those four spots. That meant he had saturated it with hydrogen; he had hydrogenated it—and he had a saturated fat now, but one that wouldn't spoil. Most of all, from his economic point of view, he had shelf life, which is what he had sought. He—and the consumer—had a fat that could not be properly metabolized.

Unfortunately, the chemical process we have just described also destroyed the essential fatty acids. Remember that we said they were essential? Well, you have to have them—but once fats or oils are hydrogenated, you no longer have them. One man once said, "Well, it's still down in there and that cell will get it out." This isn't quite true. Dr. Royal Lee, one of the most patient, knowledgeable nutritionists I have known, answered this naively hopeful statement with an analogy that's still apt. "When you take a Cadillac automobile and melt it down," said Dr. Lee, "you don't have a Cadillac any more. If you build a wheelbarrow with it, you've got a wheelbarrow instead of a Cadillac, and it will not do what a Cadillac will." I agree completely with Dr. Lee. When the saturated fat gets to that level, the cell doesn't know what to do with it. The cell is like the boy trying to put his right hand into a left-handed glove. It doesn't fit. The cell can't use it, so what happens? Usually you can count on "left-handed" substances in the body to cause trouble. The body handles the type of material it has been breaking down and absorbing for millions of years, remember. So if the cell can't use this fat that has been saturated with hydrogen, it has to go somewhere. Eventually it is deposited in the lining of the blood vessels. That's where it causes trouble, and big trouble; it's the Number One cause of heart diseases.

Most doctors recommend corn oil and their patients buy what they consider the proper brand at the store. Personally, I wouldn't let it in my kitchen, and I certainly wouldn't let cottonseed oil in, because the cotton farmer sprays every week with DDT or other persistent pesticide, which goes straight to the oil. There's no way to get it out, and it's cancer-causing. While this makes sense, why eliminate commercial corn cooking oils too? Unfortunately, most corn farmers up North spray just as zealously as the cotton farmers down South.

And there are other reasons. These common variety, supermarket cooking oils and fats have been chemically extracted. The chemical extraction method, which is uniformly used by the large commercial companies, leaves out some of the essential nutrients. It is fragmenting the natural food.

Commercial peanut oil is faulted on another score. This oil is made from No. 3 peanuts. These are the peanuts that have become rancid. When that little thin covering around a peanut is broken, the peanut will become rancid. However, the food chemists have learned how to clean it up, deodorizing and decolorizing, so that it can be sold. Profit, remember, is the guiding theme and motive in our food industry. By then it's junk, but they dress it up to look like food, and it sells as food. But it's an impostor, and should be exposed as such.

The third great offender we must avoid in our diets is

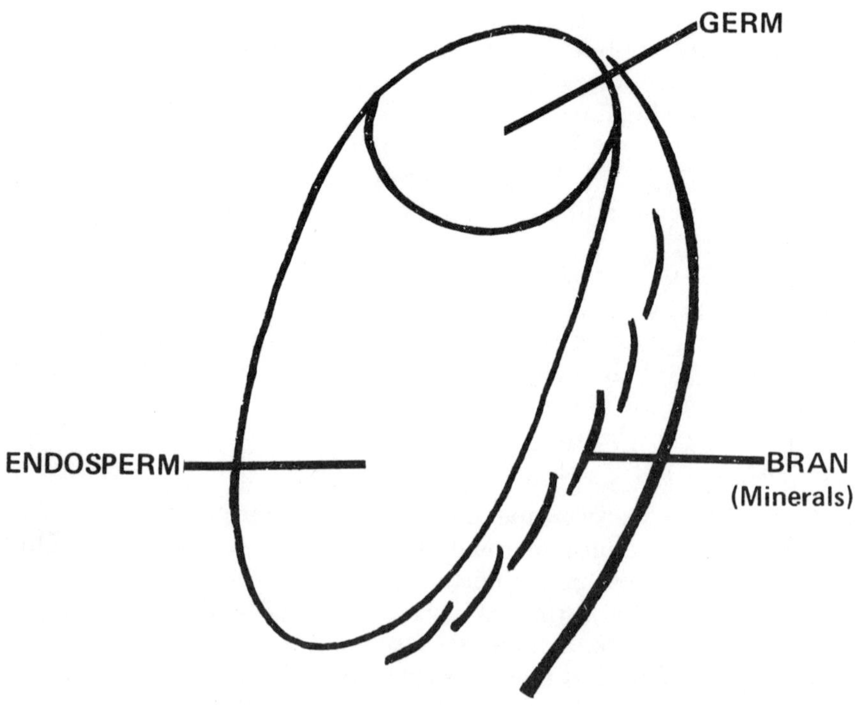

bleached white flour and anything made from it.

When I explain this to my patients, I usually draw them a picture of a grain of wheat. A complete grain of wheat consists, basically, of the germ at the end of the grain, the bran around it, and the endosperm inside. We have seen what happened to our friend who was robbed in that cold alley. This, and more, is happening to a grain of wheat during the milling process. The germ is taken out first. If the germ were left in, the flour would spoil. So they remove its life, in effect killing it now so it will not live or die later. This is a decapitation process. We ought to call modern milling the "Guillotine Process." Or the Sterilization Procedure. Next, the bran is taken out for the same reason and also to take the brown coloration out. It also takes out the minerals. This leaves the endosperm, which is starch. It is white and this gives white flour its characteristic color.

The endosperm is not quite pure starch, but it is practically so. There are some low-quality protein granules left, surrounded by connective tissue. It is nothing to get excited about, nutritionally speaking.

The best part of the wheat grain is what is taken away. The bran, in which essential minerals exist, is used for cow feed and wheat shorts that are fed to hogs. Livestock, then, get the "waste" products and are fed better than we are, if we consume white flour.

Now this is only the physical, or mechanical, part of wheat milling. Just as important from a dietary point of view is the chemical process.

The bleaching process, as if to make it whiter than snow, introduces poisons that I consider dangerous. For thirty years flour was bleached with nitrogen trichloride, which is the agene process. Dr. E. Mellanby, in the *British Medical Journal* in 1946 and 1947, reported that flour bleached with nitrogen trichloride caused running fits in dogs and some other animals. It was a central nervous system poison. The agent responsible was pinpointed as methionine sulfoximine, a by-product of the bleaching process. There was no question but that it was dangerous. On October 1, 1949, most of the millers voluntarily changed to the chlorine process of bleaching.

Other "improvers" used in flour include chlorine dioxide, benzoyl peroxide, potassium bromate, and ammonium persulfate. They did not form the poisonous methionine sulfoximine. Instead of methionine sulfoximine, chlorine dioxide bleaching produced methionine sulfoxide (note the slight difference in spelling and, therefore, meaning), as does air oxidation; no unfavorable effects have been specifically blamed on methionine sulfoxide.

However, chlorine dioxide may produce other more harmful oxidative changes in the chemical composition of flour, though none seems to have been reported. Alloxan is an oxidation product of uric acid and can be a factor in nervous or mental disorders. Hydroxypurines are relatively easily oxidized, and uric acid forms alloxan in the presence of acidic oxidants. Xanthine, a white crystalline nitrogenous compound found in blood and urine, resembles uric acid. It is more difficult to oxidize than uric acid, but alloxan has been reported as an oxidation product of xanthine under strongly oxidizing conditions involving two steps: first, xanthine is enzymatically oxidized to uric acid; then uric acid is easily oxidized to alloxan by chlorine dioxide.

Why has the presence of alloxan in bleached flour never been reported in the chemical literature? Probably because no one has ever looked for it, in order to report it. But we know that alloxan *can* be produced as an oxidation product of xanthine—and chlorine dioxide *may* be a strong enough oxidant to do it. It is quite likely that some conversion of xanthine to alloxan does occur when flour is bleached with chlorine dioxide.

Other chemicals in bleached flour may be even more harmful than alloxan. Drs. G. C. Sheldon and Allan Yorke, writing in *The Lancet,* a British medical journal, in 1953, reported the case study of a patient who developed eczema, mental disturbance, and anorexia, or loss of appetite, when fed flour bleached with either nitrogen trichloride or chlorine dioxide. The patient did not respond to conventional treatment. After several years, white flour was finally determined to be the cause of her problems. On a flour-free diet her condition returned to normal. Thereafter, a number of tests were made in which chemically untreated bread and regular commercial white bread were fed her. Each time, her symptoms returned with the regular white bread; she enjoyed normal health while eating the chemically untreated bread.

Then another interesting test was made. The patient was fed agene-treated (nitrogen trichloride) bread. She developed the expected symptoms. Then the agenized bread was withdrawn. Subsequently, she was fed bread that was bleached, instead, with chlorine dioxide. She developed the symptoms *faster,* and *all* the sites of her body where she experienced symptoms were involved within forty-eight hours and *simultaneously*. Anorexia was more profound. She seemed constitutionally more affected, looking ill, pale, drawn, and apathetic. Depression came earlier and was deeper.

In other words, chlorine dioxide, the flour-bleaching process now used, was worse for her than the discarded agene process.

The bleaching process is only part of the reason I think white flour is harmful. We have referred to the enriching process, which I have suggested could more accurately be called the robbing process. We have seen how much is taken out of a grain of wheat. The minerals and vitamins in the germ and the bran are taken out. In the enriching process they put back in synthetic niacin, thiamine, riboflavin, and inorganic iron. Niacin, thiamine, and riboflavin are merely three parts of the B complex vitamins. The natural B complex has more than twenty *known* parts. This isn't restoration or enrichment; it's fragmentation and an advertising hoax. You have to have the whole thing, all the minerals that are found in the outer coverings of the wheat germ—iron, cobalt, copper, manganese, molybdenum, and all the other natural values found there.

I am convinced that these minerals are necessary in a certain proportion to each other. I further think there is a significant interrelationship between these minerals and the vitamins in the proportions they are found in this grain of wheat. This is what I mean by balance.

The fourth item on our avoidance list is white sugar and glucose sugar. Glucose is the heavy syrup that fruits are packed in. This means canned peaches, canned pears, and fruit cocktail. Most soft drinks contain glucose. Glucose is also found in most table syrup. Glucose is corn starch treated with sulfuric acid. Most table syrup is glucose artifically colored and flavored. What a mess to put on pancakes!

The normal fasting blood sugar ought to be about 80 milligrams per cent. But when you eat white sugar and glucose immediately it goes straight into the blood stream, so that you get hyperglycemia, which is too much sugar in the blood. This excessive amount of sugar in the blood comes down to the cell. It stresses the cell, and the cell cries out, "Please, Doctor, *do* something! Somebody do something!" The cell is drowning in sugar; the pancreas hears the alarm, and the pancreas puts out too much insulin, so that you get a hypoglycemia, which is not enough sugar in the blood.

This is the physiological reason for coffee breaks. A man begins the day with a Continental breakfast consisting of orange juice that has lost all its natural vitamin C, coffee with refined sugar in it, and some commercial breakfast cereal with plenty of junk and calories but no food value. Or maybe he only had a doughnut, which has white sugar and refined flour (and hydrogenated fats), and coffee with white sugar in it. By 10 o'clock in the morning he has hypoglycemia, not enough blood sugar, because of his inadequate breakfast. This is why the factory has to shut down at 10 so everybody can get a cup of coffee or a Coke or a Dr. Pepper—which shoots the blood sugar right back up again, in a hyperglycemia state. Then again the pancreas reacts, and by noon it is way down again, in hypoglycemia. He consumes more refined sugar at lunch, and the up-down process continues, and he has to have his afternoon coffee break. This goes on all day long—at 10, 12, 2, 4, and 6. It is not only the physiological reason for the coffee break, it is also the physiological reason for sipping a Dr. Pepper at 10, 2, and 4.

The most popular soft drinks contain glucose.

He is sick at the point where his blood sugar is up, in the hyperglycemic state. Some of this sugar goes off and is deposited

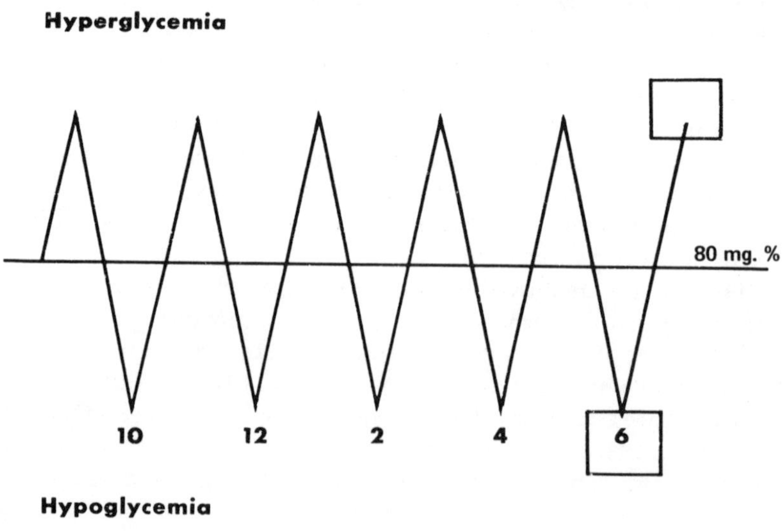

in the body as a saturated fat, which raises the cholesterol level, and is one of the causes of heart disease. But down at the point where he is in a hypoglycemic state, his resistance is lowered, he is weak, nervous, and not mentally alert. He also has lost his resistance to both viral and bacterial diseases. If he is in a state of hypoglycemia and he comes into contact with someone with a bad cold, he is much more likely to contract that cold than he would be if he were up in the normal level for blood sugar.

The only time this man is in balance is that fleeting second when he crosses that normal line.

Refined sugar and glucose are also the physiological reason for the cocktail hour, if I may be permitted to insert a bit of levity into this rather grim subject. By 6, after bouts with his blood sugar level at 10, 12, 2, and 4, a cup of coffee or a cold soft drink is not enough, so he goes by the tavern and gets himself a shot of whiskey. By the time he gets home he is feeling pretty good. It has been a long, hard day, but now he has finally made it.

But unfortunately for him, his wife is a good Methodist and she has taken the pledge, so all hell breaks loose.

The truth is that the chief cause of marital discord and divorce in America today is not whiskey, but white sugar and glucose.

Because that's what pushed him to the cocktail hour in the first place.

Number Five on our list is most dry cereals. The nutritional value of these has been so harshly and widely criticized in America during the past few years that it hardly seems necessary to go into any detail here. They are full of "empty calories." The grains used in the cereals have been degerminated and the natural vitamins and minerals removed. Then they are "enriched," but they are still so poor that leading nutritionists have indicted them as junk foods. I would add one more indictment. They are not only junk foods, they are double-junk foods, for many of them add white sugar or glucose to make them appealing to the youngsters, or even to adults.

Thus, we have come to the end of our list of the five major types of foods to avoid. I think we would have an improvement if we merely eliminated these junk foods from our diets. But it would not insure healthful eating habits. For this we need a positive dietary plan. What should we eat in place of these Five Bugaboos of the Kitchen?

The answers are as easy as counting. They are:

1. Use *unrefined* sea salt. Natural sea salt contains the trace minerals in balance. This is the essential difference between natural salt and sodium chloride. Sea salt is the best source, for it has more minerals. But remember balance. Too much sea salt would be harmful. If you eat natural foods, which contain minerals, very little salt is required. Even some of the sea salt on the market today has an anticaking agent whose safety has not been proved. Read the label! Unrefined sea salt can be found at your health food store. Vegetable salt, found at your health food store, is also safe and useful.

2. Use natural cold-pressed oils, instead of hydrogenated fats. Since we have eliminated corn oil and cottonseed oil because of the DDT content, this means cold-pressed soy, peanut, safflower, olive, sunflower seed, or sesame seed oil. At our house, we use cold-pressed safflower oil and soy bean oil.

3. Use the whole grain products instead of white flour. This means whole wheat bread and flour, which has all the minerals and vitamins left in it. Whenever possible, get this and cornmeal that is grown organically so that there are no poisons in it.

4. Use honey as a sweetener, instead of white sugar and glucose. Let me emphasize honey that has not been pasteurized, or heated. Heating destroys some of the food value. It is necessary to check closely for this. Most of the honey in grocery stores has been pasteurized. It is done for one reason, the old reason we became familiar with earlier—shelf life, so the honey won't turn back to sugar. When the honey reverts to sugar, the customer won't buy it and money is lost. At our house we use good unheated honey, which is called wild honey for that reason, not because it is made by wild bees from wild flowers.

5. Use natural unpolished rice, cracked wheat, and natural rolled oats or steel-cut oats, instead of the regular, skillfully packaged breakfast cereals we hear so much about. I do not recommend the commercial three-minute oatmeal. It has been cooked too long at high temperature, which kills the "life" in it. Fortunately, there are some natural, unrefined, untreated breakfast cereals on the market, but few of them are in our supermarkets.

When we have all this, we have the beginnings of a feast for our cell that we spoke of earlier in this chapter. With these five changes in our daily diet, we can assure a certain integrity of that cell. But, of course, there is more. We must have all of the essential nutrients that we discussed at the beginning of this chapter. One of the most important items is the protein we eat. The protein foods provide us with our eight essential amino acids, which are the building blocks of our body. There are twenty-two amino acids. Eight are called essential for the adult. Ten are necessary for the growing child. If these essential amino acids are included in the diet, the body can manufacture the other amino acids.

In America, meat is the most popular source of protein. The buying of high quality meat, however, is not as simple as once it was. Again the economic motive has intervened, between the producer and the consumer. Let me illustrate. You might say that the worst meats are the most expensive ones. The grading of beef is exactly opposite of what it should be. There are four U.S. Department of Agriculture standards of beef at present. Standard, good, choice, and prime. Prime is the most expensive and the worst. Lean meat would be graded standard—the worst grade, but the best meat.

Unfortunately, the prime steak of today comes from an animal, usually from a big feed lot, that has been force-fed for 180 days with low quality protein hybrid grains that have been sprayed with poison insecticides. This heavy fat from the forced feeding produces marbleing of the steak with a saturated fat that contains the pesticide. This type of saturated fat has been indicted as a cause of heart disease. Also, stilbestrol has been added to make the animal gain weight, and stilbestrol has been shown to be a cancer-causing chemical. This chemical additive adds nothing to the nutritional quality of the feed; it only makes the animal gain weight. Unfortunately, you see, meat sells by the pound, not by its quality.

The prime steak is the worst piece of meat in the grocery store. I grow my own beef to avoid this danger. But not everyone can grow his own meat, so the best thing to do is to buy a lean piece of meat with no fat on it. About the only place in America today where you can still get that is in a small grocery store that sells locally killed meat.

Marbleized fat has come to be something of a status symbol among steaks and roasts today, and yet it is the most dangerous type of meat we can put into our mouths, excluding mercury-contaminated fish. The marbleing makes it tender, and that appeals to us, but it also contains DDT and other pesticide residues, and it is *saturated* fat, which may be harmful to our cardiovascular systems. Eating government-inspected Prime steaks today involves taking a prime health risk.

In many big feedlots they find animals dropping dead of heart disease before they are slaughtered. These animals are obese and sick. Their livers are so full of poisons they mostly have to be discarded. The same mistake is at work here as in the sale of grains for feeds. They want the more pounds of beef, just as the farmers want the more bushels of corn, so they can make more money. Our prices are based not on quality but on production, *i.e.* monetary value.

Organ meats are good, but only if the animals are organically grown. Calves liver may be used, because the age of the animal means it hasn't had time yet to build up a residue of poisons in the liver, but all other liver should be avoided. Unless you have a source of organically grown meats, avoid chicken liver, beef liver or any other. The livers of the prime animals are confiscated, much of the time, because they contain abscesses and toxic substances of all sorts. Commercially-grown chickens have arsenic and antibiotics in their bodies and much of it winds up in the liver. The liver is the detoxifying organ in the body, and that's where these poisons go.

When I tell my patients how to approach proper nourishment for the cell, I always point out that there is a catch in it: As I have defined natural food, there's not much of it in this country. But there's enough for us, if we know where to get it.

At the present time, it's necessary for them to go to a health food store. Sometimes they are called natural food stores or organic food stores. In other places they are called ecological stores. Although most of them are limited in the basic foods, they do have quite a lot. For 25 cents, a person can get enough sea salt to last a month. They have whole grain, poison-free bread. Like much of the other natural food, it has to be kept in a refrigerator or deep freeze to keep it from spoiling. They also have whole grain rice. This is one of the best foods in the world. Orientals eat natural rice and fish, and do not develop the cardiovascular disease that we have in this country.

There is a little trick to cooking rice right. If you don't know how, you can boil it for an hour and it will still be tough. But if you take one cup of rice with two tablespoons of safflower oil and simply put it into a boiler and heat it, that oil will soak through and soften up the outside layers. Then boil that for 32 minutes, steam it for 10 minutes, and you have a high quality food. At our hospital, they call it Dr. Joe's Dirty Rice because it has the brownness from the whole grain, unpolished rice. But it's not dirty; just think of that color as vitamins and minerals, because that's where they are. Never wash it in a colander; if you do, you will wash out the B vitamins.

Another top food is the oatmeal sold in health food stores. And there's a little trick to cooking oatmeal. The best way is to soak it overnight. Take a cup of oatmeal and cover with hot water, and let it soak overnight. In the morning, you cook it for three minutes only, in the same water, because that is where the enzymes and vitamins are. If you hadn't soaked it all night, you would have to cook it 30 or 40 minutes and this would destroy some enzymes and vitamins. Once the oatmeal is cooked, put some juicy, delicious, poison-free raisins into the oatmeal, along with some honey to taste. Stir it all together. That with a piece of whole grain bread makes a fine, nutritious breakfast.

Until the day comes when Americans in huge numbers start demanding better treatment from the food industry, the health food stores will remain the safest place to buy food. I am not trying to push stock in health food stores; I have no other honest alternatives but to say that, if I am to be concerned with the health of this country. Admittedly their food stocks are limited, but they have the whole grains, grits with vitamins and minerals still intact, spaghetti and macaroni made from natural flour, stone-ground natural flour, oils, raisins, dates, prunes, dried fruits, and peanut butter made from organically grown, poison-free peanuts. Most of these stores at one time or another stock fresh, poison-free fruits that have been shipped in or grown locally. Sometimes organic vegetables are available. More and more people are turning to organic farming, so that every year we are getting an increasingly greater supply. Whole wheat or soy flour makes the best hotcakes a person ever put into his mouth. You have the added satisfaction that it isn't going to harm you but, rather, will help you. Usually cheese is available and sometimes you can find the oldtime hoop cheese and the rat cheese, as we used to call it. These are the least expensive but the best, just as we found to be true in buying the various grades of meat.

One of the best foods in the world is organically-produced peanut butter. It may or may not come with a little sea salt added. I know of no better way to demonstrate the difference between good food and junk food than with the two kinds of peanut butter sandwiches. One of the most nutritious sandwiches of all is the one made with good organically grown peanut butter spread on whole grain bread. The peanut butter, like the natural bread, has to be refrigerated as soon as the seal is broken on the jar. It still has life. It has the capacity of becoming spoiled.

But if the person takes commercial peanut butter that has been hydrogenated, he's in trouble. He's eating junk. Most of this kind of peanut butter has had a half-dozen chemicals added to keep the oil from separating (as it does in the natural variety), in order to make it easier to spread. The manufacturers brag about all this in their advertising, but when that kind of peanut butter goes on a piece of white bread, or a soda cracker, it's as bad as a person can get.

The person who feeds hydrogenated peanut butter and crackers or white bread to that cell we were speaking of at the beginning of this chapter is contributing to the ultimate breakdown of that cell and to many other cells like it in his body. Not only is he actively harming that cell, he is also starving it.

So how, specifically, do you solve this problem? What do you eat to make sure you get proper nutrition? We will be hearing more of this later on, but for the time being let me sketch out my own personal solution, to give an idea of what I eat each day, to illustrate exactly what I mean by eating right.

I think breakfast is probably our most important meal. It gets us started right, nutritionally. Forty per cent of the American people don't eat any breakfast at all, and another 40 per cent just thought they did. The man who had a cup of coffee with some white sugar in it and a sweet roll has had practically nothing that will do him any good during the day. Nor has the one who ate a piece of toasted white bread with some oleomargarine on it, an infertile egg, and a strip of bacon come anywhere close to getting proper nutrition.

When I get up at 6:30 each morning, I prepare for breakfast first by going into the bathroom and drinking a big glass of water. The pyloric valve from the stomach to the intestine is open at that time. The water will go right on down into the intestine, stimulating the peristaltic action of the intestines as well as starting the digestive juices to flowing. This helps you enjoy your breakfast more and digest it better.

I am fortunate that I live in a small city. Our public drinking water comes from 700-foot wells and is not now contaminated with DDT and other agricultural chemicals. Chlorine is used only occasionally and no poison sodium fluoride has been added to our water.

Those of you who live in cities where the water supply comes from lakes and rivers should buy bottled artesian water. This is now available in most cities.

The first thing we have at our house for breakfast is fresh fruit in season. In the fall I eat pears and apples. Then I have a piece of toast, made from whole wheat flour, followed by a couple of poached or soft-fried yard eggs. I use a little honey for sweetening and I also eat for breakfast a couple of walnuts or two pecans or about three almonds. The nut is one of the best foods in the world. Sometimes I have a couple of prunes or a couple of dates. On other days I have hotcakes with pure maple syrup, or oatmeal, or the old-fashioned Southern grits. Whatever the menu, by the time I have finished breakfast I have all the essential nutrients in balance.

When I am traveling I can pick and choose, as one can once he has learned enough about nutrition. I order melon in season. The banana is almost always available. When I order a breakfast steak I almost always have to sacrifice the potatoes they bring with it. Potatoes are good food when they are baked or boiled. But they are ruined when they are made into potato chips, and they are at their worst when they adorn a plate bearing a breakfast steak, for they are usually saturated with hydrogenated fats from frying or hash-browning. Of course I am always served enriched white bread with my meal when I am traveling. I don't say a word. I go ahead and eat the healthful part of my breakfast. Then I perform a ritual I associate with my earlier history. In my twenties I was the doctor at Dan Beard's Boy Scout camp for two summers. Dan Beard was a great naturalist and a great man. I still try to do the Boy Scout good deed every day of my life. So I just take the white bread and tear it into little parts, so they cannot feed it to anyone else.

When I am home, at noon and evening meals we have meats from our own organic farm. We have the vegetables that are in season. Since these come off the farm they are poison-free. My wife and I do our best to keep the cook from cooking too much. We tell her never to bake a pear, never to bake an apple. They should be eaten raw. We simply cut up green peppers. Cabbage and carrots are eaten raw, cut up into a slaw. We eat a lot of apple salads with pecans. In wintertime we have citrus salads at both noon and night. The vegetables come in a wide variety—beans, peas, tomatoes, squash, greens, almost every kind of vegetable that will grow in a fertile East Texas soil.

This is the stuff of which a healthy cell is made, and repaired with. Keep that cell healthy and you will be healthy.

Naturally.

VIII.
An Island of Truth in a Sea of Ignorance

Let us take a common scene about two hundred years ago. We are at a port city in England and a ship is loading for a long voyage. The ship's stores have been adequately stocked to last the long months ahead. They were careful to put aboard those foodstuffs that had "shelf life" and would not spoil until they returned to port. One food was hardtack, an unleavened bread made in very hard, large wafers. There were dried or cured meats. The food was meant to last, come storm or port. Dried beans were an almost daily part of the sailors' diet. It is not hard to see how they came to be called navy beans.

The stout-hearted sailors set sail for their destination, and at first things went well. They ate heartily and they did their work. The sea was the life, all right, and they were relatively happy and relatively healthy.

Then something began to go wrong.

The sailors developed symptoms of weakness, anemia, spongy gums, and bleeding from the mucous membranes. They had scurvy, a deficiency of vitamin C. The British sailors literally set sail on a sea of nutritional ignorance. Epidemics of scurvy hit the British navy two centuries ago and severe cases cost the lives of many sailors. Scurvy also took its toll of thousands of American pioneers who set sail for the Golden West in their covered wagons. The stout-hearted, adventuresome American empire builders were buffeted by that same sea of ignorance. Both of them started their long voyages with a food supply that had "shelf life" but little vitamin C.

The British navy started adding fresh limes to its stores, which solved its scurvy epidemics, by providing vitamin C. Today such epidemics of scurvy are no longer to be feared. However, Americans today are breezing over a similar sea of ignorance, and in many instances many are drowning in it. This is because too many Americans believe a number of myths, widespread and popularly accepted, regarding nutrition.

Myth: America is the best fed and the best nourished nation on earth.

The Truth: There is no doubt that America is overfed and overnourished. Obesity is one of the greatest nutritional problems facing America today. And the basic cause of obesity is too many calories. Foods that contain only empty calories account for the major portion of the diet of too many people. White sugar and glucose, our daily bread and the many products made from white flour, the modern dry breakfast cereals and the hydrogenated fats are directly responsible for thousands of obese individuals. The delicious, delectable, death-dealing desserts made from these empty calorie foods are known to be responsible for dental decay, cardiovascular disease in almost everyone past the age of twenty, and many other metabolic diseases. The truth is that America is the most fed and the worst nourished nation on earth.

Myth: Very few conditions or diseases are caused by dietary deficiency. "Tired blood," a feeling of being "run down" or experiencing fatigue is rarely, if ever, due to faulty diet in this country.

The Truth: It is difficult to understand how anyone with ordinary intelligence could make such a preposterous statement. Yet this is a direct quote from an article that has appeared in two national magazines. True enough, the author was not a doctor. But the magazines have been highly respected by a large number of readers. I suppose the term "tired blood" refers to the condition usually called anemia. Our pediatricians see thousands of infants who are anemic and they routinely give these babies vitamin and mineral supplements. Iron deficiency anemia is perhaps the most common form encountered, but other trace minerals, including copper, cobalt, and molybdenum, are known to play an etiological role in this disease. Vitamin supplements, including the B complex vitamins, vitamin E, vitamin C, and others, are now known to be necessary in the proper treatment of many of these cases.

It is true that frank fulminating beriberi and scurvy are no longer common in this country. These extreme deficiencies are rarely seen simply because our doctors and even most laymen now know that proper diet plus proper vitamin and mineral supplementation can and does prevent these formerly fatal diseases. Epidemics such as occurred in the British navy are no longer to be feared. But mild cases of scurvy are still epidemic in America. Symptoms of mild scurvy usually unrecognized by too many are loose teeth, bleeding gums, petechial hemorrhages, and a tendency to bruise easily. Many cases of Vincent's Angina, pyorrhea, and peridontal diseases are really due primarily to malnutrition, chiefly a deficiency of vitamin C.

Recently I saw a sixteen-year-old boy who had been treated energetically for two weeks with antibiotics and oral antiseptics. The diagnosis was Vincent's Angina or trench mouth, proved in the laboratory. He was getting progressively worse. When I saw him he could only swallow liquids and this with difficulty. He had profuse bleeding from the gums, which were reddened and edematous. I deliberately stopped all medication and gave him large doses of vitamin C. We gave him fresh orange juice, natural vitamin C complex, and intravenous ascorbic acid. Within twenty-four hours he was eating well, and in three days he was dismissed from the hospital. This was an extreme case, but we see scores of mild cases every month in our practice. Doctors all over the country who are trained properly in nutrition see and treat thousands of these cases every day.

Ninety-eight and five-tenths per cent (98.5%) of Americans have dental caries. Peridontal disease is rampant. Refined carbohydrates, sugar, and glucose are known to be primary causes. These empty calorie, devitalized foods form a slime on the gums and surface of the teeth. This slime is a perfect breeding ground for pathogenic bacteria. This microcosm along with a dietary deficiency that leaves the host no resistance quickly results in both dental caries and peridontal diseases.

The prevention of dental caries is simple. Avoid refined carbohydrates, which include white sugar and glucose. Get proper nutrition by eating only natural, poison-free food grown on fertile soils. Get as much fresh fruit and vegetables as possible and do not overcook any food. Then keep your mouth clean. This can be done with a good scrubbing on a daily basis with a soft toothbrush using salt and soda. Many dentists add a bone meal supplement to help prevent dental caries.

What a more effective and safer solution to dental caries is this than artificial fluoridation of the public waters! Sodium fluoride, the poison used in fluoridating water supplies, is a far-out solution that does not work. There is no way under the sun to control the individual dose of sodium fluoride in the public water; athletes, diabetics, and manual laborers will drink more than what is alleged to be the therapeutic dose. Furthermore, sodium fluoride is believed to have an injurious effect on the ill, the elderly, and probably others. In NFA we believe artificial fluoridation of public waters to be nothing more than "scientific" pollution.

In recent years we have learned that not only dental caries but cardiovascular disease, diabetes, arthritis, gallstones, and kidney stones are what we term metabolic diseases. These diseases are caused by what the late Dr. Tom Douglas Spies called a chemical imbalance in the body. And these diseases are rampant in America today. We are still wallowing in the same sea of ignorance that engulfed the British sailor. In too many instances we have found a small grain of truth and we have misused it. For instance, it was found that certain vitamins would relieve certain symptoms. The modern chemist was able to synthesize the so-called active principle. This pure crystalline chemical was added to some of our devitalized foodstuffs. This scientific method was supposed to be a great breakthrough and the health of our people was to be "enriched." Unfortunately, a little knowledge is a dangerous thing. The enrichment of so many common foods with synthetic vitamin A and D has resulted in a hypervitaminosis that is doing untold damage to our infants. The chemical imbalance in their little bodies has been made worse.

A number of years ago while I was vacationing in Mexico, I was surrounded by a swarm of Mexican children, each asking for a nickel from the American tourist. But I was curious and I made a counter-proposal.

"I'll give you a *peso* each," I said, "if you'll show me your teeth."

The Mexican *peso* is worth 8 cents in U.S. money. They were quite willing to go along with the strange American.

So I looked into the mouth of every Mexican child there. It

was a revelation. Each one had perfect teeth! How many American children in a group like that would have had perfect teeth? However, when you reflect on the situation, it is easily understandable. Those Mexican children were eating tortillas made from yellow cornmeal—natural food grown on fertile soil—instead of white bread. The rest of their diets was probably comparable. That was a number of years ago and they hadn't yet got into the habit of drinking soft beverages loaded with glucose. Since then the American way of nutrition has hit Mexico and I'd be doubtful if I could find so many perfect teeth in such a group like that again.

A short time ago I had quite a different experience than I had that day in Mexico. I was speaking at the University of Texas at Austin to a group of about 250 persons, predominantly students.

I asked them, "How many of you have all your teeth and no fillings?"

A couple of persons held up their hands.

"Well," I said, "we're all sick." Then I asked, "How many of you eat soda crackers?"

The hands flew up.

Then I asked, "How many of you know what is in a soda cracker?" and none did.

"You're not only sick, you're ignorant!" I said. "I guess we'd better get an education."

In the process of our educational session I was asked, "What is the first step toward having a heart attack?"

"A hole in your tooth," I said. "You've already taken the first step."

He said, "Doctor, I guess you misunderstood my question. I was referring to heart disease."

"No, I didn't misunderstand you," I said.. "The same thing that causes a hole in your tooth also causes heart disease."

They too had believed the myths of American nutrition, and they too had already got some early symptoms of heart disease. I outlined for them a program of proper nutrition. There and at other university campuses where I have appeared across the country, the young people have become very concerned about their health and about the poisons in their food. There and at other campuses I have suggested that if they really want to help build a strong America and if they like to march—and many of them do—they should march down to a bakery and surround it and just demand a good loaf of bread. Peacefully, of course. The greatest need in this nation today is for a good loaf of bread—and a cracker that won't kill you!

The way bread is made commercially now, and for the past few decades, it can be truthfully said that half a loaf is worse than none.

Myth: Americans have to go out of their way, nutritionally speaking, to avoid being well nourished.

The Truth: Americans have to go out of their way to find poison-free, high quality food. Devitalized, overprocessed foods are found in abundance at any supermarket. Refined carbohydrates and hydrogenated fats fill the shelves. The precious natural vitamins and minerals so necessary for good health have been removed from most of our bread and cereals. The essential fatty acids found in natural oils have been destroyed by the process of hydrogenation. Heart attacks and strokes are the inevitable result of this mad "scientific" process.

The truth is that America is not well nourished but is only over-nourished with over-processed, devitalized foods. These over-processed foods not only offer little more than empty calories, they are also the most expensive foods in America today, the food ads' claims to the contrary. A good example is the box of rice cereal that is a best seller. A box of it contains only four ounces net weight but sells for 23 cents. That amounts to 92 cents per pound for rice that has had its vitamins and minerals removed. The consumer is being forced to pay for the robbing procedure. In many instances, the natural, unrobbed food does cost more, but I would rather pay 50 cents for a good loaf of bread than pay 25 cents for a worthless loaf of white bread. The difference you save in doctor, hospital, dental, and drug bills will more than make up for it.

We are all still paddling in the sea of ignorance, but slowly the waves part here and there. As chief of the Health, Education, and Welfare Department's nutrition program, Dr. Arnold Schaefer conducted a survey of the nation's health in 1969. His survey shocked the scientific community and government officials. It need not have shocked anyone acquainted with the NFA story. Deficiencies of vitamins, minerals, and protein were found in all age groups, in all economic classes. Rich people, he discovered, eat the same kind of devitalized food that poor people eat. Affluence, poverty, whatever the material state, malnutrition was rampant. This made it official. It was nothing new to those of us who have been concerned for long years. We already knew America was sick.

Yet as a nation we are still sailing across that sea of ignorance, and I am speaking of all levels of our society. Even professional medical men take their daily dips into that metaphorical body of enervating water. As a result, the subject of proper nutrition is not taught in our medical schools.

Recently a new medical school was organized not far from where I live. The first class had thirty-four students, and the ultimate goal is to graduate 100 doctors, many of whom will be family doctors who can help fill the great need for physicians in our general area. One of the professors from the new school visited our medical society. He explained the difficulties of organizing a school, and he asked our help and cooperation in the school's growth.

When he finished speaking, he asked if there were any questions.

I have never been shy about asking questions, at least not in recent years, so I said, "Yes, Doctor, I have one. Are you planning to teach nutrition at the new medical school?"

"Why, what a foolish question!" he quickly answered. "Why, of course."

"Who will be the head of the department?" I wanted to know.

"We are not going to do it that way," he said. "I am the professor of my specialty, and I will teach nutrition in my specialty. Professors in other specialties will teach nutrition in their specialities."

I didn't pursue the subject any further publicly then, but after the meeting I found him alone.

"Doctor," I said, "do you let children eat crackers?"

"Why, of course."

"Doctor, do you eat crackers yourself?"

"Why, sure I do—don't you, when you have soup?"

Then I said, "Doctor, do you know what is in a cracker?"

"Well," he said, "it has flour and—"

Well, as it turned out, he was not sure just exactly what was in a cracker. I didn't say anything else. I was determined to be the diplomat. But I thought to myself, How tragic this is; the professor who is going to teach nutrition to a group of young medical students doesn't even know what is in a cracker, much less know what the ingredients of that cracker will do to the human body.

One of the leading brands of crackers, selling for 40 cents a pound, contains only five ingredients: refined salt, hydrogenated shortening, white flour, a little degerminated rye, and soda. Five cents worth of junk food, selling for 40 cents. And practically everything that goes into it causes heart disease.

If I had to pick out one item in the American diet as the worst, and crusade against it, I would choose the cracker.

As discouraging as it was to hear the professor of medicine make this statement, I can understand why he knows so little about the foods we eat today. The sea of ignorance is large enough to contain everybody. Twenty-five years ago I knew as little as he, and if I had not become a victim of heart disease I probably would still be eating crackers. I went through medical school without learning much about nutrition. I had been taught that America was the best fed, healthiest nation on earth, and I thought we had an abundance of good food. In my book, white flour, white sugar, and oleomargarine were good for health. I only hope the good doctor-professor is able to swim out of the sea of ignorance less dramatically than I had to.

It is not uncommon for a medical man to push back the waves of ignorance as a result of a personal experience. Dr. James Greenwood, Jr., clinical professor of neurosurgery at Baylor University's College of Medicine in Houston, told a scientific symposium how his golf game was being destroyed by a back disc problem that also brought him severe lumbosacral pain. But he had read somewhere that vitamin C would help his condition, and he started taking large doses of the vitamin. The pain disappeared. He resumed his golf game. Then, as an experiment, he stopped taking vitamin C. The back pain returned. Next, he resumed vitamin C therapy. The pain again vanished.

He mentioned his experience to a friend, Dr. Paul Harrington, a widely-known orthopedic surgeon. Dr. Harrington said he was also using vitamin C in his patients with back trouble and had had good results.

Dr. Greenwood made no claim that vitamin C could be considered a panacea in the treatment of back disorders, but he thinks vitamin C therapy is at least "a factor in the disc problem." In an article published in the *Medical Annals of the District of*

*Columbia** he wrote that "Vitamin C is important in the maintenance of proper texture of teeth, bone cartilage, blood vessels, and connective tissue throughout the body." Unlike the British sailors of an earlier day, we know that vitamin C is necessary in body metabolism. But even now we still know very little about how or why it is essential.

Dr. Greenwood was perceptive in trying vitamin C, although many other doctors would have pooh-poohed his experimentation with vitamin therapy. Vitamin C, after all, is a water-soluble vitamin and does not build up in the body; therefore, there was no risk in getting too much of a good thing. And citing the words of Albert Einstein that "the accumulation of knowledge only further reveals the hopelessness of knowledge or understanding more than a small bit about the universe," Dr. Greenwood told the symposium of scientists in 1964, "With our increasing knowledge, the understanding of the intricacies of the chemistry of the body becomes more hopeless. This does not mean that present knowledge should not be used to its greatest extent, but it does indicate that one should not be forced to wait for complete scientific knowledge before using methods of treatment which are *not harmful* and which show hope of success."

Dr. Greenwood followed his own advice in selecting vitamin C therapy to cure his painful back. And on the basis of simple common sense, anyone following Dr. Greenwood's precepts would logically have to apply them to natural, poison-free food. Even those strongest defenders of refined foods would not, I think, claim that natural foods are harmful. And the evidence is already in that they do promote and preserve health.

When I say natural food is the key to nutritional success, I am revealing a whole grain of truth. In too many instances, we are still wallowing in our sea of ignorance because we have found a small grain of truth and have misused it. A number of years ago this occurred in a scientific experiment that, instead, became a chapter in the story of fragmentation. I should say a "scientific" experiment, for the practice of science is as prone to error as is the programming of computers. Possibly computers are nearly free of error, but if an error, even a small one, is programmed into one, then the computer magnifies it ten fold, perhaps a hundred fold, and perpetuates it. This can be seen in one experiment per-

*Vol. 33, No. 6, June, 1964.

formed by the U.S. Department of Agriculture at Ithaca, New York. It is part of another great myth.

Myth: Commercial U.S. agriculture treats soil as a precious commodity and keeps it rich through crop rotation and fertilization. Even if our soils were widely impoverished, this would *not* mean that foods grown on them would be nutritionally inferior.

The Truth: Proponents of this myth would have you believe that a carrot grown on poor soil is just as nutritious, ounce for ounce, as one grown on fertile soil. They would have our farmers and ranchers believe that poor soil grows just as good grass as fertile soil, and that the only difference is quantity. They would have the farmer believe that the fertility of the soil has nothing to do with the quality of food grown on that soil. But we in NFA believe that poor soil grows poor food that makes poor people who are sick.

Those accepting the myth base their views on the Ithaca experiment I have just mentioned. When it was completed, the experiment demonstrated that it does not matter if a soil is fertile or not, as far as quality of the food grown on it matters. The only difference between poor soil and fertile soil, according to the experiment, is that fertile soil grows more of whatever is being produced. Higher yield, then, but of equal quality.

This is really an astounding piece of information. It assaults one's sense of logic and common sense. But before we accept or dismiss it, let's take a closer look and try to examine its scientific basis.

Here is the way the experiment was done. The USDA took an old, worn-out farm near Ithaca and divided it in half. On one half they did nothing except plow and plant. On the other half they added recommended applications of NKP, the usual commercial fertilizer consisting of synthetic nitrogen and acid-treated phosphate and potash. This was the experiment. The NKP-splashed side was classified as the fertile half; the other was the poor land. Then when the foods had been harvested, they conducted a very careful, accurate, scientific analysis of the produce, comparing each side of the farm.

Do you know what they found? This: no significant difference in the vitamin, mineral, or protein content of the two sections. Careful examination of the milk from cows grazed on the competing acreages showed no significant difference. They concluded that the fertility of the soil had no influence on the quality of food grown; only the quantity was increased. The experiment was reported in the *Journal of the American Medical Association.* In due time it became enshrined as "scientific evidence" that, even if our land is poor, the food is still of good quality.

Of course, it proved nothing of the kind. The logic behind this is specious. And it was an incomplete experiment and therefore unscientific. Furthermore the results were misinterpreted and applied much too broadly. The experiment was valid, but the aims of the experiment were misstated. What the experiment did prove was that commercial fertilizer will grow a poor quality food no better than that produced on poor land. If the researchers had claimed no more than that, there would be no argument. There *could* be no argument.

The scientific approach would have been to divide the farm into three, instead of two, sections. They should have handled the first two sections just as they did in the experiment: nothing added on Site No. 1, but commercial fertilizer applied on Site No. 2. Then Site No. 3 should have been built up like any experienced organic farmer would enrich his soil. Then the produce from the three sites should have been carefully analyzed. This would have taken into consideration the value of trace minerals and organic matter. It would have demonstrated that the mere addition of ordinary commercial fertilizer does not restore the fertility of the soil. And it would have shown what fertile soil really is.

Hopefully, such an accurately-conducted experiment would have served as an example for thousands, perhaps millions, whose thinking has to some extent been influenced by the publication of that incomplete experiment. One highly-publicized example of misguided science can, like a hurricane in a real sea, multiply the dangers already present in the sea of ignorance. One such article can do much to undo the lifelong work of someone like Sir Albert Howard, who more than fifty years ago proved the relationship of the fertility of the soil to the health of both livestock and people. Dr. William Albrecht of the University of Missouri has spent a lifetime proving the simple, vital truths of soil fertility. The late Dr. E. E. Pfeiffer proved in his laboratory at Spring Valley, New York, the superiority of the quality of foods grown on fertile soils. The Pennsylvania Dutch, the Amish, and thousands of organic farmers all over America know that fertile soils result in healthy livestock and a healthy people.

When we find ignorance so rampant among our better-educated people, it comes as no surprise when we find "nutrition blanks" among the rest. I have encountered it day after day in my own practice of medicine.

One day a Negro man brought three of his children into my office. He had ten children in all, and they were always sick. Their health problems ran a gamut from runny noses and runny ears to fractured bones. They were just sick all the time. His wife was dead and he was ready to leave. I knew he didn't have much money. I thought I could help him. I asked him to sit down so I could tell him how to feed those children so they wouldn't be sick all the time.

But he said, "Well, Dr. Joe, I haven't got any money, and I can't buy that expensive food." He had already heard about "Dr. Brown" and his diet, and he had the idea it was strictly for rich men.

"Well, sit down anyway," I said, "maybe I can help." After he had sat down I continued: "Have you got any hickory nuts out there in those woods behind your house?"

"Yes sir," he said. "The woods are full of hickory nuts."

"You don't eat them?"

"No sir."

"Well, next Saturday afternoon, why don't you get your children to go hickory nut hunting? Remember how you used to do that when you were a kid? Get you a couple of grocery sacks and fill them up. Then bring in the hickory nuts and you'll have enough to last all winter."

"Well, I hadn't thought about that," he said.

This was the fall of the year and I said, "You got any pecan trees?"

"Oh, yes sir," he said, "down at the old house place, there are a whole bunch of pecan trees."

"Have you eaten any pecans?"

"No sir."

"Well, go down there and get a bunch of those pecans, pull them in, put them in your house, hang them up. Hang up a winter's supply just like a squirrel would. You got any pear trees out there anywhere?"

"Oh, yes sir, we got some pear trees right in our backyard."

"Do you eat any pears?"

"No sir, we don't like them."

"You got any persimmons out there anywhere?"

"Oh, yes sir, the woods are full of persimmons."

"Do you ever eat those?"

"No, they pucker your lips."

"What do you do, just let the coons and possums eat them?"

"Yes sir."

"Well, when they're ripe they're soft and sweet and don't pucker your lips. Why don't you get you some traps and stay out there and catch some of the coons and possums? That's good meat. And you eat those persimmons. They're not going to hurt you. They're good for you."

"Well," he said, "I hadn't thought of that."

Here was a man who had all these natural foods at his back door. He had worlds of proper nutrition that was free to him, and he didn't know it. He too was swimming in a sea of ignorance. The tragedy is, his is not an unusual case. There are many of us, even in cities, who could have a backyard garden and grow our own delicious, poison-free vegetables. And there are millions of Americans who every day buy the wrong kind of food because they don't know how to read the labels and don't know how various foods are processed. And there are many others, like the patient I just told about, who overlook the bountiful nutrition that is theirs practically for the asking, or getting.

If we are to survive, all America must be educated to the dangers we now face and must be told how we can avoid the national disaster we are headed toward. Modern scientific agriculture is an assault on nature, an ecological blunder, and is destroying mankind. Modern scientific infant nutrition with its emphasis on calories and its ignorance of quality is destroying the health of our babies.

The American people have become almost resigned to their fate. To many, the situation is hopeless and they have all but given up in what should be the prime of life. After fifty, one must die of something! Good health after fifty is not expected by most Americans, and good health before fifty is unusual in most Americans.

Even doctors are floundering. The average physician and dentist in this country knows very little about proper nutrition. He eats crackers and junk food just like everybody else, and he dies with heart disease, cancer, and diabetes just like everybody else.

But all is not lost yet. There is an island of truth in this vast sea of ignorance. It is good and beautiful, and it is simple. It is the NFA story. Natural, poison-free food grown on fertile soil, eaten fresh, and not overcooked.

IX.

In A City Apartment

Tim and Debbie had been married a year when she had her miscarriage. They lived in one of our large cities. Tim was twenty-four, out of college a year, and holding a good job as an accountant for Universal Paper Shufflers, Inc., a wholesale business. He and Debbie had met at the Midwestern campus where both of them had graduated. Debbie, twenty-three, was a legal secretary for one of the vigorous young legal firms in the city.

Debbie's miscarriage came during her second month of pregnancy. She had hardly had time to discover she was pregnant before the miscarriage happened. Scarcely had she begun adjusting to the fact that she was to be a mother, than she lost the child she and Tim had already started talking about and planning for. The loss left her empty emotionally and she even felt a tinge of guilt. Maybe more than a tinge. She and Tim wanted two children. It seemed they were starting out wrong.

For a couple who had started out their married life so full of exuberance and optimism, things seemed to certainly be going poorly. They had thought they had their whole lives ahead of them. The miscarriage was like a slap in the face from fate. Then close on the heels of Debbie's miscarriage, other assaults came from the same fate. Tim's allergies got worse. He started sneezing uncontrollably; hay fever kept his nose running so much it seemed he spent half of his day just blowing and wiping his nose. Sometimes he got headaches. He went to an allergist and got an elaborate set of tests. The allergist, noting some of his allergies were due to certain foods he ingested, put him on a diet. The allergist checked a list of foods, complete with brand names, that Tim should avoid. He started administering regular injections to combat the allergies. Tim began to improve, but at twenty-four he had been made painfully aware that he was sick. If it had been just he, it wouldn't have been so bad. But Debbie, now over her miscarriage, continued to have menstrual cramps; on many days she just didn't feel well. It was more than her having the blues over losing the foetus. She felt lousy.

One thing they both had in common. They both felt especially lousy in the afternoons. Neither one could hardly wait until the first coffee break after lunch. Tim usually could get away for a cup around two or three p.m. Sometimes Debbie was busy taking dictation or typing a transcript and was lucky if she could have some coffee brought in. Those days, she felt terrible by time she got home in the afternoon.

One day Debbie read something about natural foods. A girl friend of hers she worked with in the law firm showed her an article in a magazine called *Natural Food and Farming.* Debbie was not interested in farming, whether it was natural or unnatural. She, like Tim, was urban born and urban bred; she had never been closer to a farmer than the lettuce and potatoes in the supermarket. But she liked her girl friend and out of politeness said she would take a look at the article. Debbie knew her girl friend went a little overboard about "health food stuff." She would even have called her a "health food nut," except that they were good friends. It's hard to call a friend a nut. But the friend was a little way-out about eating, it seemed to Debbie; after all, food was food, wasn't it? I mean, what's the difference, as long as you get the different *types* of basic foods you're supposed to eat? Anyway, that health food stuff was high; Debbie had gone to a little place down the street for lunch one day with her friend and they had drunk carrot juice and she had priced some of the stuff they had on the shelves. But Debbie felt terrible all the time now and she promised she'd take a look at the article.

She read the article that night and thumbed through the rest of the magazine, and she told Tim, "Maybe this man's got something. Why don't you read it too?"

The article told about how America's food supply is sprayed

with pesticides, nurtured with synthetic fertilizers, and then overprocessed until it wound up a dangerous, overadvertised, debilitated hoax on the consumer's table. The author wrote of specific instances when risky chemical additives were put into food. He mentioned some diseases that were associated with a number of the fragmenting procedures through which America's food supply went.

Tim read the article with furrowed brow.

"You know, maybe he's got something," he said.

"Well, Kitty thinks so. She's a real nut about natural food. But she always seems to be so *healthy*. She's *disgustingly* healthy."

"Maybe that's why," said Tim, nodding at the magazine.

"She never has a headache. She never has trouble with her period. And she seems so . . . radiant, all the time."

Tim and Debbie decided Kitty's way was worth trying. They read *Natural Food and Farming* from cover to cover that night. They even examined the yellow pages, with the directory of natural food dealers throughout the United States. They noticed that one natural food store in their city advertised therein.

"But how do you get started? How do you know what to do? How do you know where to buy and what to buy?" said Tim.

They both knew they were sick, even though they were in their early twenties. The more they thought about it, they realized they weren't really as happy as they'd kept telling themselves they were. How could anybody be happy when he or she was sick?

Debbie talked with Kitty at length the next morning during the coffee break. Debbie had skipped breakfast again and was having her usual coffee and doughnut. Sometimes she varied the routine, and ate a jelly roll. Sometimes she just bought a cola drink out of the machine down the corridor. Kitty usually drank a fruit juice.

Debbie asked Kitty whether she ever went to a doctor. Then Kitty told Debbie about her doctor. He was a "Dr. Brown" in that large city. Unfortunately, said Kitty, there are not many physicians at the present time who rely on natural, poison-free food as the best medicine, but there are some. She gave Debbie her doctor's name. She suggested Debbie and Tim get an appointment with him, to have him brief them on proper nutrition. Kitty was smart enough to know that an enlightened man with an M.D. degree would probably impress them more deeply than she could.

Besides, she thought "Dr. Brown" might be able to give some specific prescriptions for Tim and Debbie's specific health problems.

Tim and Debbie went to see "Dr. Brown." He was a warm, kindly man who seemed deeply interested in what they said. Kitty had told them he was a member of an organization called Natural Food Associates. Tim told him about his allergies and his treatment; he mentioned his headaches and told how he hardly ever felt very well. Debbie explained about her miscarriage and how they later hoped to have children. She explained she was back on the Pill for birth control purposes. As had Tim, she told him how she seemed always to be run down and out of energy.

"I see," said Dr. Brown. "What do you have for breakfast?"

Debbie smiled a little nervously.

"We don't always eat breakfast," she said.

Dr. Brown smiled.

Debbie said, "Sometimes I scramble eggs with bacon. Maybe we'll just have toast, buttered—"

"Real butter?"

"With margarine. And maybe orange juice."

"Canned juice?"

"Yes."

Tim said, "A lot of times I don't have time for breakfast. If I'm hungry I'll eat something at a cafe close to the office, later in the morning."

Dr. Brown said, "But you always have a coffee break?" His eyes glanced from Tim to Debbie.

"Never miss one," said Debbie. Tim's smile told the doctor the coffee break was a ritual with him too.

Dr. Brown next questioned them about their lunch, then dinner, and soon had a clear pattern of their dietary habits. He also learned they got very little exercise during the course of a day. They rarely got out of the city, except to another city, or even to any of the several spacious parks in their own city. He learned that their nutritional education went little farther than knowledge of the basic foods they had learned in school, plus what they had read in the one issue of *Natural Food and Farming*. Then he handed each of them a mimeographed "health sheet."

Debbie's eyes skimmed over the health fact sheet. Dr. Brown listed in one column the food products and the additives they should avoid. These included hydrogenated fats, refined sugar and products using it, refined salt and products using it, white bread and white flour products, and foods with chemical additives. He warned about certain foods, such as vegetables and fruits that were not organically grown. Carrots, for instance, if not organically grown were probably sprayed with pesticides. The danger, though, was not from pesticides on carrot tops but from poisonous residues that remain in the ground and were taken into the root by the carrot. The couple was warned to peel all fruit that was not organically grown, to avoid ingesting pesticides such as might be on the peel of an apple.

In another column on Dr. Brown's health list, the couple was told what to substitute for the foods they should avoid. These included cold-pressed natural oil and fats, organically produced peanut butter, honey, whole grain breads and flour, and foods without chemical additives.

"But where can we get all these?" asked Tim, a little bewildered by now, but charged with enough knowledge to be anxious to find safe food.

Dr. Brown told him. He explained that they would have to educate themselves to the dangers of modern shopping, that health factors were just as important as cost and taste when they were buying for the kitchen and table. It would help if they continued regularly to read publications that would keep them informed and up-to-date on foods and the environment. He named a number of stores in the city where they could buy a number of natural food products. He mentioned one that was an outlet for organic farmers in the area, from which he himself bought fresh, organically-grown vegetables. He suggested the couple inquire at the natural food stores about ordering fruit and vegetables from organic farms and that they check advertisements of such farmers in the publications they would be reading.

The doctor also suggested that the couple embark on a regular program of exercise, such as jogging in place or even jogging down the street and around the block, and that they do it together. He suggested that each of them use their two automobiles only when necessary and use their feet and legs more. Avoid elevators when they had to go up or down just a few floors. Never ride when they could walk. He suggested parking several blocks from their work so they would build that much exercise into their daily routines. And he recommended weekends in the country or at the park, with lots of walking and communing with nature. He also suggested that they take up a game or a sport, such as golf, that they could participate in together.

He emphasized the importance of breakfast. Even if it meant getting up thirty minutes or more earlier each day, he said, they should both have a leisurely, substantial breakfast with natural, poison-free foods. They should find a source of fertile eggs and poison-free fruit. He showed Debbie how she could vary the breakfast menu and get off to a radiant start each day.

The doctor told them how to buy meat, when they had to depend upon the grocery store and the supermarkets for their supply. Ignore the grading labels that have been placed on the meat, he said, and buy the cut that has the most lean on it and is not marbleized. Avoid meat of any kind that has fat on it, because the pesticides store up in the fat. This pretty well eliminated pork, which is higher in fat than any other type of meat. They were told never to eat beef or chicken livers, never to use chicken necks.

"But what about restaurants?" said Tim. "Can we eat out once in a while?"

"Sure," said the doctor. "But become accustomed to knowing, automatically, what is good and what is dangerous. Know, without thinking, not to eat the white rolls and bread. You can always do without bread for one meal.

"If you're ordering breakfast, order eggs poached so hydrogenated fats won't be used to cook them. Ask for real butter and accept no substitutes; do without it, if necessary. Order a breakfast steak.

"Stay away from the delicious, delectable, death-dealing desserts. Finish the meal with fruit if you can. If you're eating at a cafeteria, choose the freshest looking foods. Beware of the way a food may be dressed up and think about what it is and how it has been prepared. If you're ordering in a restaurant, stay away from items you know are dangerous, such as French-fried potatoes and pizzas made of white flour, and try to order a good lean steak or baked or broiled fish—a good protein source—and, if possible, a good distribution of fresh vegetables or fruits."

Before they left that day, "Dr. Brown" gave Tim and Debbie a reprint, "Read That Label!" by Beatrice Trum Hunter, to help guide them in their safaris to the supermarket.

"Dr. Brown" also gave them a copy of instructions he gave his patients for the dietary management of heart disease. He pointed out that although neither of them exhibited what might be considered clinical symptoms of heart disease, it was a danger faced by almost everyone in America today and, besides, if they approached their diets as if they *did* have heart disease, they would solve most of their other health problems too.

After they got home that day, Tim and Debbie carefully looked over the material he had handed them and several phrases and paragraphs that the doctor had told them began to ring through their minds.

"Never eat a food that will not spoil, but eat it before it does. This is a cardinal principle that must be obeyed if one expects to get proper nutrition."

"Most Americans overcook their foods. Heat destroys vital nutrients. A steak should never be well done. It should be cooked medium rare. The best restaurants will not take an order for a well-done steak. This not only destroys the vital nutrients, but it also destroys the flavor. One exception to this rule is pork. Unless pork is well cooked, it may cause trichinosis."

"White sugar and glucose are known to increase the blood levels of cholesterol. Corn starch is treated with sulfuric acid to form glucose, a synthetic sugar. This sugar is rapidly absorbed into the blood, causing a hyperglycemia, which is followed within hours by a hypoglycemia. This empty calorie 'food' causes a rise in the blood cholesterol and must not be included in the diet of the atherosclerotic patient. These synthetic sugars are found in canned fruits, most bottled soft drinks, candies, cookies, and table syrup."

"We also exclude white sugar because it has been so refined that it too contains no vitamins or minerals. Since we increase the caloric content of the diet with natural oils, we exclude all empty-calorie foods possible."

"Until you can find natural, poison-free foods in sufficient abundance, you may have to resort to supplements. Vitamin F tablets (essential fatty acids) are available. A natural multivitamin tablet and a natural vitamin E tablet after meals are recommended."

"Administration of synthetic multiple vitamin and mineral tablets advertised so highly over radio, television, in newspapers, from door to door, and in drugstores is not a satisfactory way to insure proper nutrition."

And they remembered these specific dietary instructions:

1. *Bread*—Only whole grain breads freshly ground and made without chemical additives should be used.

2. *Sweets*—Untreated honey is the best sweet. Old-time ribbon cane and sorghum syrup is good. Real maple syrup is a delicacy.

3. *Cereals*—Natural, unpolished rice contains all of the essential B vitamins and is one of our best foods. It is almost as good as the wild rice of Minnesota, and is less expensive. Cracked wheat and natural, unprocessed rolled oats found in health food stores are also good foods.

4. *Oils*—Cold-pressed natural oils are essential to good health. These are the most difficult of all natural foods to obtain in America today. Safflower, sunflower seed, and sesame seed oils are good sources of the essential fatty acids. Cold-pressed soybean and peanut oils are available. Most commercial cottonseed oil and corn oil contain too much DDT to be recommended.

5. *Vegetables*—Use fresh, poison-free vegetables grown on fertile soil. Eat a green and a yellow vegetable every day. Raw vegetable salads are best. Cabbage should not be cooked. Heat destroys vital nutrients.

6. *Fruits*—Use fresh, poison-free fruits in season. Eat the whole fruit, not just the juice. Wash and peel commercial fruits. This will *not* eliminate all the poison. Poison spray residues are vitamin antagonists and enzyme inhibitors. Organically grown poison-free fruits are now available in limited supplies.

7. *Eggs*—Fertile yard eggs are best. They should be poached, soft boiled, or lightly scrambled in natural oil or good butter. Most commercial, infertile "caged eggs," produced with poor feeds to which antibiotics have been added, are of poor quality.

8. *Dairy products*—Good butter is permitted. It is a natural food and contains vital food nutrients. The fats in good butter have not been artifically hydrogenated. Unpasteurized natural cheese is also permitted. Exclude pasteurized milk unless there is no source of fresh, raw Grade A milk.

9. *Meats*—Eat lean beef and lamb and do not overcook it. Cheap cuts of meat usually contain less marbleized fat. Use organically grown meat and poultry if available. DDT accumulates in the fat, and residues of stilbestrol may be found there. Do not eat commercial chicken livers. They may contain arsenic.

10. *Nuts*—Fresh nuts are permitted. Do not eat too many.

When they got home that day, Tim and Debbie inaugurated

a revolution. They signed their own declaration of independence. They declared themselves independent of the tyranny of advertising and packaging. They resolved never to let themselves be beguiled again by the slick promises of the food advertisers on television, never to buy a product because of the way it was wrapped or packaged or advertised as a bargain or the way it was advertised with tantalizing adjectives. They decided that day that they had a right to enjoy proper nutrition, that it was one of their freedoms that they had almost lost, and that it was as important as any of their other freedoms.

Debbie's first revolutionary action was to clean out her apartment's kitchen. She threw away the refined salt. She dumped the white sugar and the white flour she had on hand. She took the hydrogenated cooking oil and the oleomargarine and she discarded it. She put the bread they had on hand and the two frozen pizzas into the garbage. The crackers and the (hydrogenated) peanut butter went. She read the label on the syrup they had been using, and she got rid of it. Systematically Debbie went through the items in her cabinet, refrigerator, and shelves. Everything that was on the "avoid" list she discarded. She read the labels, even the minute print. If there was an ingredient that she didn't understand or had a long chemical name on it that she couldn't pronounce, it went.

When she was through, she and Tim surveyed the refrigerator and cabinet shelves—and laughed.

They had to laugh, because there wasn't enough left to make a decent meal.

And they were hungry.

So they went out to a restaurant and each ordered a medium rare steak with mixed green salad and a baked potato. They trimmed off the fat, ignored the white rolls and manmade "butter," and passed up the dessert on the menu. But they did have a dessert—the restaurant had fresh bananas.

Then they went shopping, first at a natural foods store they had heard of, and then to the supermarket to get a few things they could buy there.

To their surprise, the total cost was about what they usually spent for groceries, even with the two steaks added in!

It was not easy at first to break old habits of eating and buying that they had carried with them all the way from childhood. They had to find substitutes that were healthy when they wanted something sweet, rather than eating ice cream or mellorine from the supermarket. Debbie learned how to make her own ice cream, using raw honey and fertile eggs. But the more they read and learned, the more they discovered that, far from limiting them in diet, their nutritional horizons had been widened. For the first time, they began to actually *taste* their food, and they added a new dimension to living.

Debbie, remembering what "Dr. Brown" had told her about interfering with the natural processes of the body, also stopped taking The Pill as a birth control measure, and she and Tim returned to mechanical means of contraception. But even this kind of birth control would be only for a limited time, for both mates did want to start a family sometime in the near future.

Now after what "Dr. Brown" had told her about the dangers to the foetus because of items in the American diet, she was glad she had learned this and had changed her dietary habits before she got pregnant again. Next time, she would not miscarry.

In a short time, Tim and Debbie were living a vastly different life in their big city apartment. They had never realized they could have found so many natural foods, as cut off as they were from the land. Tim's allergies receded, then practically vanished. He still remained under an allergist's care, but even the allergist was impressed at how he had improved. Now both Tim and Debbie felt good nearly all of the time. Her menstrual cramps lessened and seemed on the way out. They both felt fine in the afternoons.

Six months after seeing "Dr. Brown," at a time when she felt physically and emotionally vibrant and was ready for it in every way, Debbie learned she was pregnant again.

X.

And Baby Makes Three

Tim and Debbie were jubilant. Debbie was going to have a baby! They would be parents. This time, there would be no miscarriage. Despite the previous miscarriage, despite the fears that had come out of the first ill-fated pregnancy, Debbie felt exuberant. Both she and Tim were optimistic this time. Most of all, they felt confident, confident that she would carry the child to term, confident that they now would be able to do everything possible to insure that the baby would be born healthy and whole.

When her obstetrician informed her she was pregnant, Debbie returned also to "Dr. Brown" for special dietary instructions for her pregnancy.

Although she by then was on proper nutrition and, therefore, had been preparing her body for the pregnancy, her visit to her dietary specialist, as she had come to think of this physician whom we have called "Dr. Brown," reemphasized certain elements of her diet that would now be exceedingly important.

The most important time in the life of a child, biologically speaking, she was told, is from conception until birth. During those nine months, the baby's body is being formed so rapidly that deficiencies of certain vitamins in certain stages can cause birth defects. It is also known that mental retardation is much more likely to occur in children born to malnourished mothers.

The doctor pointed out that there was adequate scientific proof of these facts in the medical literature.

Therefore, the doctor told Debbie, if a mother wants to have a good healthy child she ought to get on proper nutrition herself at least six months before conception. This gives her a healthy body to start with. Then if she eats properly the chances are excellent that she will deliver a normal, healthy baby.

The doctor smiled. It pleased him to note that Debbie *had* started a program of proper nutrition at least six months before her and Tim's baby had been conceived. This provided an extra glow of satisfaction for the parents-to-be.

By Debbie's being on proper nutrition, the physician pointed out, she had pretty well insured her baby from being born with one of the severe health problems that are attacking the very young in America today: birth defects, rampant cancer, diabetes, dental caries, even heart disease by the age of three!

The next most important time in the life of a baby, Debbie was told, is from the time of birth until one year. Here, again, the baby is growing very, very fast, and it is tremendously important that he get proper nutrition at this particular time of life, because if he doesn't, damage may be done that will remain for a lifetime. Damage at this point cannot be repaired, and there is adequate proof of this.

The foundation for strong bones and good teeth and a healthy body is being formed in this extremely important time of life. Perhaps at no other time in life, after delivery, is it more important that the child get all the essential amino acids, all the natural vitamins, the necessary organic minerals, and the essential unsaturated fatty acids.

Unless the baby is breast fed, he has very little chance of getting proper nutrition. If the mother has had a good diet, containing all these essential nutrients—barring accidents—the baby usually is born into the world healthy and ready and able to nurse the breast.

There are two general lines of reasoning as to why a mother should breast feed her baby. One concerns the positive benefits of nursing, so that the baby gets exactly the nutrients, in proper balance, that nature intended. There is no way under the sun that man can duplicate mother's milk. This is worth repeating and thinking about. No laboratory has done it. No laboratory is likely to do it. A weak substitute, perhaps, but that is all.

On the other hand, there are the negative features, the risks and damages incurred by *not* breast feeding. Anything that is not breast feeding must be called artificial feeding. In cases where artificial feeding must be resorted to, there are some methods that are more desirable and more health-oriented than others. Those suggestions will be taken up subsequently.

But what are the risks involved in artificial feeding? Here are some of the points that Debbie's doctor discussed with her.

Atherosclerosis, the forerunner of heart attacks and strokes, begins in infancy. Recent studies from 1,600 autopsies revealed fatty spots in the aorta of many children under three years of age and *in all children over three years of age.* Coronary artery fatty lesions are almost always present in persons over the age of twenty.

The cause of atherosclerosis has been fairly well proved in recent years. Refined, free-flowing salt, hydrogenated fats, white sugar and glucose, and white flour products are implicated. Modern baby foods contain refined, free-flowing salt.

Until recently monosodium glutamate was added to baby foods. This chemical has been implicated as the cause of the Chinese Restaurant Syndrome and the cause of brain damage. The Chinese Restaurant Syndrome refers to the symptoms of headache, dizziness, and muscular pains after the patient has eaten a Chinese meal in which monosodium glutamate was liberally used to add flavor.

Modern canned baby foods cannot give the baby proper nutrition. Not only is it fragmented and inappropriate to the needs of the child at that particular time, but frequently brings risks we often learn about when it is too late. The tragedy is that the baby foods industry has also been tainted by the spectre of modern American chemical agriculture.

Several years ago, scientists at the University of Missouri found 40 parts per million of nitrate in a two-ounce jar of both beets and spinach. Anything above 12 parts per million of nitrate *per day* is considered toxic to an infant. Nitrate poisoning is very, very common in this country today.

We have had "crib deaths" by the tens of thousands in this country. Little babies go to bed apparently healthy and then are found dead. These crib deaths have long puzzled physicians and researchers. But Dr. Barry Commoner, professor of botany at Washington University, has suggested that nitrate poisoning may be one of the factors in these crib deaths. It is not the only cause, but it may be one factor.

We have known for a long time that nitrate poisoning causes "blue babies." The nitrate combines with the hemoglobin to form methemoglobin. Methemoglobin cannot transport oxygen; therefore the baby turns blue. One of the first cases reported was that of an infant in Iowa that was delivered normally in a hospital. The baby went home, was put on a formula, was given water from the family well, and the baby turned blue. The mother ran back to the doctor with her baby. By the time she got to the doctor the blueness had cleared up, and the baby was apparently all right. So the doctor thought that it was just a case of a nervous mother. But the mother took the baby back home, gave him another formula made from the same well water that had too much nitrate in it as a result of extensive synthetic nitrogen fertilizer on the farm, and the baby again turned blue. The same course of events took place. She rushed the baby to the doctor, but its blueness had cleared up by the time she got to his office.

Finally, she kept feeding the baby the same formula with the same water, and the baby turned extremely blue and was still blue when she got him to the doctor. Fortunately, this was a very sharp doctor, and he recognized the symptom as one of nitrate poisoning. They tested the well water. It was very high in nitrate. It was what we call a "hot well;" it was hot with nitrate. The family subsequently got a good, healthy source of water. They solved their baby's health problem. Fortunately, they discovered the trouble before losing their baby, for other babies have died of this.

The farmers of America, through ignorance, had been poisoning little babies!

How else can you put it? That family in Iowa had a close call as their baby got an overdose from a hot well. But other babies in America, who don't live close to a farm, also have received their own toxic overdoses of nitrate, from the residues that have accumulated in baby foods produced by farmers using commercial fertilizers.

Well, if the baby is not breast fed, or is being weaned, what does the mother do? Debbie by now had already decided she would breast feed, but she wanted to know what to do in case it didn't work out.

Until refined salt, monosodium glutamate and excessive

amounts of nitrate are removed from our baby foods, the doctor told her, the young parent has but one choice. She must get a blender and buy poison-free foods from the health stores for her baby. She should buy the foods she would eat herself and then run the food, just as she would eat it, through the blender. Then feed it to the baby just as it comes from the blender. As soon as the baby can handle solid food, she should feed him off the table. Once she starts that, she won't be able to make him eat baby food because he won't like it.

Most of the time, breast-fed babies are fed too early. I personally do not think they should be fed anything but breast milk until they are at least three months old. I don't think the digestive tract is ready for food that early, and I'm quite sure that many allergies result from feeding too young.

At six weeks we usually put breast-fed babies on orange juice and cod liver oil for supplementary rations. We shun the synthetic vitamins that babies usually are given. If a baby is breast fed, the mother doesn't have to start feeding him until he is at least three and a half or four months old. But if the child is not breast fed, it is important to start feeding him a little earlier, for the chances are he is not getting what he should get out of his formula. This may mean getting a blender and beginning his feeding career at three months. Proper nutrition at this early stage of life can't be overemphasized, for a child on poor nutrition doesn't have resistance to diseases; he gets both viral and bacterial infections, colds, tonsillitis, ear infections, and any number of viral diseases that tend to run in epidemics.

But without a doubt, the first choice of mothers in caring for their infants should be to breast feed. The advantages of breast feeding are once more becoming apparent to both the mothers of America and to their doctors. For too long, both mothers and doctors have been content to feed the babies from a bottle filled with canned milk, synthetic sugars, and synthetic vitamins. Many formulas have been made available in liquid and powdered form that are supposed to be "almost identical" to mother's milk. In many areas, fewer than one-third of our babies are breast fed. There are many reasons for this deplorable condition. Women have gone into industry in large numbers; they no longer have time to nurse their babies. In some areas of our society, the mothers have become convinced that it is neither "fashionable" nor "scientific" to nurse the baby. They have come to believe that modern scientific infant nutrition means artificial feeding. Even some of our best medical authorities in the field of pediatrics have said there is no longer any nutritional advantages in advising breast feeding.

Oberman and Burke have stated that it is a sad commentary that a large segment of the opposition to breast feeding arises in physicians and hospital personnel who are unwilling to take the time to educate and instruct new mothers on the advantages and proper methods of breast feeding a new baby. Some physicians, however, still insist on breast feeding and are willing to spend the time and effort in educating the mother to the benefits due both her and the baby. But the majority of physicians—and this includes too many pediatricians—either don't know the difference or sincerely believe that it makes no difference whether the infant is breast fed or is artificially fed. The whole subject of nutrition has been badly neglected in our medical curriculum. Infant nutrition, perhaps the *most* important branch of nutrition, is the most neglected.

The simple truth is that there is no comparison in the values of mother's milk and artificial feedings. The breast-fed baby gets the essential nutrients in the proper proportions, just as lactating mothers have provided for their offspring since the dawn of man. Every mammalian species naturally produces the right formula for its babies. Mother cows, goats, dogs, horses, and elephants produce exactly the right kind of milk for baby cows, goats, dogs, horses, and elephants. Each "formula" of each species is a little different from the other, because the needs of each are different. The same is true for humans. Human babies need human milk. Nothing that a laboratory cooks up, no matter how well advertised and popularized by Madison Avenue, will change these human needs worked out by nature over the hundreds of thousands and millions of years. Cow's milk—even raw Grade A cow's milk—is not the same as human milk. Cow's or goat's milk, if untampered with, may be the next best thing to human milk, but it is not the same and cannot do the job as well.

All of the nutrients that the breast-fed baby gets in proper balance, the result of untold generations of human development, are lost to the bottle-fed baby. Artificial feeding contains a few synthetic vitamins which, to put it mildly, are of dubious value. The usual carbohydrate added to the formula is also a synthetic sugar that does not maintain a normal blood sugar level. The milk itself has been processed and pasteurized and heated until the vital life factors, so necessary for good nutrition, have been destroyed. True enough, the artificial feeding may make the baby fat, but a fat baby is not a healthy baby. The growth and development of the breast-fed baby is not only superior, but this baby is more resistant to both infectious and viral diseases. That is one of the natural roles of human milk. If the mother is told that her baby will be much less likely to contract polio if he is breast fed, she usually will cooperate, and it is true that breast-fed babies who continue to eat from a table of natural organic foods are practically immune to poliomyelitis. Breast milk contains valuable antibodies that cannot be duplicated in an artificial formula.

There are many other advantages to breast feeding, the doctor explained to Debbie, even though by now she was sold on it. He pointed out there is less danger of bacterial contamination. Breast milk is obviously less expensive, and it is easier to prepare. Infantile eczema is less frequent in breast-fed babies. Allergic conditions are increased sevenfold in artificially-fed infants. The mental health of the child begins with the proper mother-child relationship in infancy, and this means breast feeding.

There are also some important advantages to the *mother* who nurses her baby. The young mother with her first baby has usually gained from twenty to thirty pounds in weight. Her whole body has been covered with a deposit of fat. She has lost her girlish figure. This layer of fat was added for a purpose, to help feed the baby. The nursing mother gradually loses this fat and regains her girlish figure without difficulty. But the mother who is given stilbestrol injections to "dry up" her breast will find it much more difficult to lose the excess fat.

The modern mother can make a choice. She can eat natural food of high quality and nurse her babies: they will be healthy, and she can maintain her youthful figure with normal healthy breasts. (Breast-feeding mothers tend to have a lower incidence of breast cancer too!) Or she can eat devitalized empty calories and feed her child an artificial formula that can only lead to early metabolic disease in her child—while her "dried up" breasts, injected with stilbestrol, provide fertile soil for cancer.

In concluding his advice to Debbie, the doctor quoted Eberle's 1834 statement: "There is no substance in nature, nor can there be anything prepared by art, which forms so congenial and wholesome a nourishment, during the period of infancy, as human milk."

In order to give Debbie added encouragement and to provide a regular source of information and communication with other breast-feeding mothers, "Dr. Brown" suggested that she join La Leche League (9616 Minneapolis Ave., Franklin Park, Ill. 60131), a non-profit, non-sectarian organization that offers help "to all mothers interested in good mothering through breast feeding." The doctor informed Debbie that there was a La Leche League chapter in her city, as there are in many large cities today, and he urged her to get in touch with it. He also prescribed that she read *Nursing Your Baby* by Karen Pryor or *The Womanly Art of Breast Feeding,* the official book of La Leche League, or another good book on breast feeding.

The story of Debbie and Tim is a never-ending one, because it is one that grows and grows with the years, like the story of any young couple concerned with proper nutrition and willing to go to some trouble to attain it for themselves and their children. As the years pass by, other problems present themselves. So it was with Tim and Debbie.

In the post-weaning years of childhood, Debbie zealously saw to it that her child was fed properly. This was easy to do, for Tim and Debbie ate properly themselves, and to feed the youngster was only a matter of feeding him what they ate themselves. For a while, until he had fully functional teeth, it was necessary to grate apples or to shred organic carrots. Sometimes Debbie concocted a fine meal for him with her blender, putting in vegetables or fruits. She found a source of Grade A milk. By the time he was ready to eat anything from the table, there was no problem. It was just a matter of serving him a child's portion.

But Tim and Debbie's family was growing. A couple of years after Tim, Jr., was born, Debbie became pregnant again. By then they were thinking about larger living quarters. They would have to find a larger apartment, to accommodate two youngsters, or they would have to buy a house. They decided to buy a home. They had been considering this now for another reason, so the decision came easily when they learned definitely that Debbie was to become a mother again.

The home they found would give them enough space for all the family. Best of all, it had a backyard. The backyard was one of the items Tim and Debbie scrutinized most closely when they looked at a place they might buy. They didn't demand a huge one, but it had to be fairly large, if at all possible. Of course, they wanted enough room in back for the children to play. But they also wanted enough room to make their own garden there. Tim and Debbie had grown up in the city. They had spent all of their married life in an apartment. They intended to continue living in the city. They were urban people. But they wanted their own garden. If the Japanese could grow vegetables in the tiniest of plots, why couldn't they?

During the pre-school years their children's diet was no problem for Debbie. Then suddenly, as Tim, Jr., started to school, parents Tim and Debbie realized they faced a new problem, in regard to nutrition. Tim, Jr., and then later their daughter, Sarah, would be leaving the bosom of the family nutritionally even if it was for only one meal a day. What should they do?

By this time, Tim and Debbie knew enough to figure out solutions for themselves. They were armed with knowledge. They were sophisticated, certainly as pertained to nutrition. And like any good researcher, they began solving their problem by first collecting all the facts available to them.

What about the school cafeteria where Tim, Jr., would eat? In May of the year Tim, Jr., would start to school, his parents visited the school and ate at the school cafeteria. They discussed the menus with the teachers and the school dietician. They did not tell their own views; they merely collected information, and they carefully observed all the foods that were served and how they tasted and how they were prepared.

They were not favorably impressed with their meal, despite the glowing reports from both teacher and dietician as to how much the children loved the food. But Tim and Debbie were tactful and only smiled. After all, they had not come there to argue with sincere, honest, conscientious operators of the cafeteria, but to gather data that would be helpful in making their decision.

For days Tim and Debbie debated the school diet problem. They had also observed that soft drink machines were available in the hallways of the school, even for the first graders! And they could buy potato chips and candy bars and other junk foods. Although the presence of these machines was depressing to Tim and Debbie, they were primarily concerned with the quality of the food served in the cafeteria. Their children, having been reared on natural food, might not be tempted to buy junk food and drinks from a coin machine—but he might have to eat in the cafeteria.

What should they do? What could they do?

Tim and Debbie turned the problem over and over, looking at it from every side. They finally decided, despite the overwhelming, popular belief held by teachers, administration, cafeteria personnel, children, and other parents, that Tim, Jr., (and, later, Sarah) could not get proper nutrition from the school cafeteria as it was then set up. But would one such meal a day hurt, when he would be getting proper nutrition at breakfast and the evening meal and on weekends and during summer vacation? Well, the noon meal was an important one. Over a period of time, a considerable load of chemical additives would be consumed. If he ate bread there, it would be white bread. Peanut butter there would be hydrogenated peanut butter; sometimes it was made into peanut butter cookies—hydrogenated fats supplemented by white flour and white sugar! If Tim, Jr., were given a list of things to avoid in the cafeteria, he wouldn't have much left to eat. And he would seem odd to the other kids. This is important to a youngster, and Tim and Debbie didn't want him to get self-conscious about food in the presence of his age peers.

It was appealing to think that, even if Tim, Jr., did eat at the school cafeteria, he would be getting only a fraction of the junk food that the other kids would be getting. But still, agreed Tim and Debbie, he would be eating junk food. It would not be fair to him. They just would not feel comfortable with his eating there.

They talked again to one of the first grade teachers and casually asked if any of the children brought their own lunches to school. To their surprise, they found that some did. Probably not for the same reason Tim and Debbie were considering it, but the fact that it was done by some would not leave Tim, Jr., standing out like a sore thumb.

They decided Tim, Jr., should take his lunch. Debbie was determined to each day fix such a good and attractive lunch that Tim, Jr., would be proud to show others how much his mother loved him by making him such an appealing meal. The other kids would be envious. How could Tim, Jr., be criticized for carrying his lunch then? Each day he opened his lunch box or paper bag in the cafeteria where he would eat with his fellow first graders, he would be able to enjoy a minor cornucopia. There wouldn't be anything oddball about that, would there?

But that fall, when school started, Tim and Debbie realized they were confronted with a long-term educational program. The other parents, to begin with, had to realize the children weren't getting proper nutrition. But this had to be presented subtly. Tim and Debbie realized this. They also had to diplomatically alert the cafeteria personnel to some of the dangers in the kitchen. From time to time, Debbie would drop by and chat with the dietician about something she had read and would clip an article about nitrates and nitrites in food. In this way she was able to have commercial hot dogs taken off the menu. She had made friends with the school dietician and was not arrogant with her knowledge, and therefore the dietician had read the information with open mind. Bit by bit, she began to have an influence and was in a position to offer the dietician a free subscription to *Natural Food and Farming* or other health publication.

There was much, nutritionally speaking, that could be improved about the school. Tim and Debbie felt that since their children would each be attending classes in the school system for twelve years—or a total twenty-four years for both of them—they were obligated to do what they could to improve the "health environment" of the school.

The physical education program of the school was fine. They liked the teachers who were dedicated, hard-working men and women. It was a well-run school and the city had fine schools where Tim, Jr., and Sarah would attend after they had finished elementary school. They had no quarrel with the curriculum. But like most other schools in America, the nutritional environment left something to be desired.

There were two areas in which Tim and Debbie thought they might be able to do something: in the cafeteria, and the vending machines. They had made a start in regard to the cafeteria when Debbie made friends with the dietician. But it was also essential that they also make friends with other parents and get them interested too. Tim and Debbie joined the Parent-Teachers Association (PTA) and regularly attended meetings. After they had been in PTA for a while and had got to know the others and learned to like them, Tim and Debbie diplomatically (oh, so carefully!) brought up the matter of the vending machines. They didn't call it "junk foods," but they quoted enough from well-documented medical articles to demonstrate that such soft drinks and candies cause dental caries. These parents could proudly proclaim by then that neither child of theirs had a single carie. No other parents in that school, that they knew, could claim that. Tim pointed out that the public schools of Altoona, Pennsylvania, under constant encouragement from Dr. Fred Miller, had banned pop machines. It was not difficult for Tim to find a dentist who was willing to speak to the PTA group on the dangers of "pop" to dental health, especially in children.

This young couple was most perceptive in realizing that people can be changed toward an intelligent point of view but that it must be presented patiently and with extreme tact. A man or woman does not want anyone to say he's stupid or dumb. So they did not say any of these things. At no point were they insistent or strident or self-righteous. They respected the views of anyone who opposed their opinions, even though the opposing opinions represented everything they were against. In this way they helped build a spirit of mutual tolerance that encouraged everyone to consider the pros and cons without undue emotion or pressure of projected personal threat. Tim and Debbie did not push anyone into a decision to take out the drink and candy machines over the emotional reactions of the businessmen who had put them there. But by calmly, patiently presenting the facts and letting the others make up their own minds in an atmosphere devoid of stress, Tim and Debbie had an influence even ten times their number might not have had, an influence that would in time benefit thousands.

We have to end our endless story somewhere, so let us say that Tim, Jr., and Sarah grew healthy and learned and became good citizens, and Tim and Debbie lived happily ever after, all quite naturally.

XI.

Let's Grow a Garden

Back in the days when I was recovering from my heart problem and slowly learning, by reading and by experience, what it meant to eat natural, poison-free food grown on fertile soil, I also began learning how to grow a garden that would provide proper nutrition.

It was a trial and error experience, and sometimes laughable, as I look back on it today. I was so sold on the virtues of organic fertilizer that I overdid it.

In the late 1940's when I returned from the convention of the American Nutrition Society, I was, as I have already confessed, a "real, sure-nuff goin' joker." I was not only going to save the world, I was going to set the first example and in the grandest style. I had a 1,000-acre farm there in East Texas, but I started my actual gardening and farming operations on a one-fourth acre plot. On this garden site I was determined to have the most fertile quarter-acre this side of the moon.

At least I was going to have the best garden in Cass County, Texas. I was convinced that the organic way of farming was the only sensible way. In my enthusiasm I set out to excel the first year. I had the organic matter—cow manure from the barn and lot—and I had the land, and I had the exuberance and confidence.

"Clean out the barn," I told my farm manager. "Put all the manure on the garden."

No more commercial fertilizer would ever be used on Jonica Farms! It was like setting off on a new adventure, or a new life.

My farm foreman did as ordered. Good barnyard manure would enrich the soil if anything did.

One day the foreman called and said, "Well, Dr. Joe, I've cleaned out the barn and put it on the garden."

"Good," I said. "How much did you have?"

"Twenty-seven wagonloads," he said, dead-pan.

Twenty-seven wagonloads of cow manure on a one-quarter acre of land!

We went ahead and planted the usual garden with tomatoes, squash, carrots, and all the other vegetables common to our part of the country—the works, in other words. But, of course, my first organic gardening experience boomeranged on me. There was too much manure. The vegetables couldn't even stand up. There was too much manure and not enough soil. I had overfertilized and had "burned up" my crop. I had overdone a good thing.

I had made the greatest gardening mistake one man could make. This turned the garden into a dust bank. I should have spread the twenty-seven wagonloads over five acres, instead of a quarter acre. Nonetheless we had learned a vital lesson. Most people still think that if a little is good, then more is better. But I learned dramatically that year that balance is the secret. I was to learn that balance in all things is essential to a contented, healthy life, whether it is in food, farming, or life generally. You can take too many vitamins, you can eat too much good food, you can work too much, you can play too much. Without balance, life and health both get out of kilter.

Thank God, I learned my lesson early. The next year I moved the garden site—I had plenty of land—and went at my organic gardening in a more balanced fashion. That year I had a fine garden.

How did I do it? Well, it isn't an elaborate secret, and the formula applies whether you're operating a large truck-gardening plot or a simple, small backyard vegetable garden such as our friends Tim and Debbie had at their home in the big city. Here's a blueprint of gardening that you can fit into your own life, whether you have a spacious, unused meadow or a tiny backyard site.

SITE

Choose a fertile site that is well drained and can get sufficient sunlight. If possible, do not choose a plot where commercial fertilizers and poison insecticides have been in long use. Do not choose a site too large. Tailor the size of the garden site to the size of your family. You can grow all you need on a small plot. Properly cared for, the produce from a half-dozen tomatoes, squash, and okra plants will surprise you. A handful of bunch bean seed has supplied enough green beans for numerous neighbors as well as the family that planted them.

PREPARATION OF THE SITE

The soil should be plowed in the fall. Do not use the moldboard plow to "turn under" the litter in the topsoil. It should be "disked" in. On larger plots the chisel plow is best. Composted animal manures should be applied and disked into the soil in the fall. A rototiller is best for the small garden.

COMPOSTING

A compost pile should be started. All kitchen wastes, leaves, grass cuttings, and any other such organic matter should be piled together in some vacant corner of the yard or near the garden site. Some topsoil, raw rock phosphate, and rock potash may be added to make a better compost. The use of a bacterial activator will speed the process and limit any offensive odors. Animal manures of all types are much more valuable when they have gone through a compost pile. *Never* use raw animal manures of any kind on your garden. I recommend *Soil And Health* by Sir Albert Howard for specific details on building a compost heap.

In these days, you can find compost already sacked, if you live in the city. Most chain grocery stores in America sell dehydrated cattle, sheep, and chicken manure, and some comes from cotton burrs, pecan hulls, and bark of trees. All these are satisfactory for composting. The feedlots of America have a problem in disposing of their manures. Of course, the proper answer to this problem is to compost it and put it back onto the land. The vast chicken industry is another source of manures. We use chicken litter, composted; a bacterial activator with forty-two strains of bacteria is simply applied to a pile of chicken litter, which is turned two or three times. This method makes compost within three or four weeks, ready for the garden.

Another thing that is becoming more available in this country (and it is being used extensively in Europe) is the composting of garbage from cities. Instead of going into the lakes and rivers, where the municipal sewage causes serious pollution, it is composted, sold, and put back onto the land. This solves two problems at one time, and indicates an area that needs much more investigation in this country.

COVER CROPS

In October, plant a green cover crop of legumes. The seed bed should be rough or in furrows so that the ground will be properly aerated. Plant only one-half of the garden in the cover crop. Save one-half for planting an early garden.

PLANTING THE EARLY GARDEN

Many farmers plant onions, cabbage, beets, lettuce, and carrots in the last days of December and early January, depending on which part of the country they are in. The "old twelve days"—in the Christmas season—is the best time to plant an early garden.

PREPARATION FOR PLANTING

The green cover crop must be disked in at least six weeks before the garden seeds are planted. The compost should be applied and disked in with the cover crop. Green manure crops are a temporary shock to the soil and must be completely decayed before planting. The insects will devour your plants unless you follow this rule. But the cover crop is invaluable. They put God-given *free* nitrogen into your soil, plus large amounts of organic matter.

IMPORTANCE OF MICRO-ORGANISMS

You must have a fertile soil if you expect to have a successful garden. This means a soil in which the conditions are optimum for the growth of soil micro-organisms. A fertile soil is a living soil. The soil micro-organisms are the "chefs" that feed the plant, the doctors that produce the natural antibiotics that give us healthy plants. They are the bridge over which the minerals get into the plant. Therefore, anything you do to help the soil micro-organisms is right, while anything you do to harm these organisms is wrong. They live on organic matter. They eat it continuously, for breakfast, dinner, supper, and for in-between meal snacks as well. So the one most important ingredient of your garden should be organic matter. Organic matter is ten times better if you compost it first.

FERTILIZERS

We never use synthetic nitrogen or acid-treated rock fertilizers, which are the ordinary commercial fertilizers. These acid fertilizers eventually destroy the soil micro-organisms and even the earthworms. Earthworms are indispensable in a fertile soil. But the acid in commercial fertilizers is dangerous to earthworms and the smaller micro-organisms and in time kills them. Even if the acids did not kill them, in time they would perish from lack of nourishment, for commercial fertilizers do not contain the nutrients that earthworms and micro-organisms must have in order to survive. Such acid-treated commercial fertilizers, then, are not only poisonous to the earthworms and the "chefs" of the soil, they are inadequate as food to this beneficial soil population.

Commercial products that contain only the raw rock fertilizers in a composted organic matter are available in 50-pound bags. They are no more expensive than the acid-treated fertilizers, and the garden requires less and less of them each year, instead of more and more, as in the case of the usual commercial fertilizers.

CONTROL OF INSECTS

Books have been written on this subject, and it may seem presumptious of me to dispose of it in a few paragraphs. Simply stated, though, plants grown on well-balanced, fertile soils do not have the same attraction for insects as those grown on poor soils that are artificially stimulated by acid-treated fertilizers. This has been proved beyond question over and over by successful organic farmers. Fertile soils have a natural immunity to insects and disease, just as a properly nourished body has a natural immunity to disease. A person can grow both quantity and quality food by using the same methods that were used before deadly insecticides like DDT and Malathion were discovered and used indiscriminately.

Certainly in the beginning some insects will probably appear in your garden. But these can be controlled by the old-time pre-World War II pesticides that our fathers used. Rotenone, pyrethrum, Black Leaf Forty, ryania, and sabadilla dust are potent insecticides, but used according to directions they are safe. These pesticides come from plants themselves, and within two or three weeks after application they break down into nontoxic materials. By harvest time, they are no longer toxic, but the postwar chlorinated hydrocarbons and phosphorous insecticides that Rachel Carson warned of in *Silent Spring* do not break down for years, as we all well know today. We also use diatomaceous earth with pyrethrum in many cases.

Some organic farmers buy useful insects, such as the ladybug, and earthworms to put into their gardens. I have never done this, because I had them all over the place. If you make the conditions optimum for the growth of soil life, the earthworms will come from somewhere. If you plant some flowers in your vegetable garden, bees and other helpful insects will come even more. The ladybugs that will come are among your best friends. Welcome nature's allies. They will make life easier, and safer, for you. If not mistreated, nature always leaves a little bit left over, whether it be the eggs of useful insects or of earthworms. Nature, treated like the queen she is, provides the biological controls.

MULCHING

Organic gardener Ruth Stout has written a book, *How to Have a Green Thumb Without an Aching Back*. She uses a heavy mulch of leaves or grass or straw to prevent the growth of weeds and to conserve moisture. This is a highly successful and specialized method. But I would suggest that you get her book before adopting the method. There are some pitfalls. Another excellent book is *Gardening With Nature* by Leonard Wickenden.

You can grow a garden, and you can have fun doing it. The principles I have outlined in this brief blueprint are the same, regardless of the dimensions of your garden site. You may live in the country and have unlimited choices of site and size, or you may live in a city shared by millions and have only a small postage-stamp backyard. But you can grow your own vegetables and possibly have fruit trees in either type of environment. You may not be able to grow all your vegetables, but even a little is very helpful. Besides, the exercise is good for you. It will contribute to your health and your happiness, and it will not cost you. It will pay you. What other reasons do you need?

XII.

Timely Changes for Changing Times

In the 1940s I was faced with converting a worn-out, 1,000-acre East Texas farm into a fertile, organic farm. It was as near completely worn-out as you could find a piece of property. It had been cropped in cotton and corn for years, and nothing takes the rejuvenating life out of the soil like those two crops.

By then I knew something of organic methods. I had been reading and I had learned by personal experience through my quarter-acre garden. But the rest of the large farm was a bigger problem than a mere garden. I called the county agent, and we drove down to the farm. I wanted his help in making a decision as to what to do. The county agent came equipped with shovel and cans, in order to get a soil test.

As we arrived at a field, I asked him how much a soil test would cost.

"One dollar each," he said.

"How many are you going to make?" I asked.

"About ten."

"That's going to cost me ten dollars," I said. "I don't see any use of wasting that ten dollars. I think anyone can look at that land and tell that it needs everything."

He laughed.

"Doctor," he said, "you are a scientific man, and you know the scientific way to determine soil needs is to make a soil test.

We send it down to Texas A&M College and they analyze it and get the Ph, and analyze it for organic matter and for nitrate, phosphate, and potash."

"Yes, I know that," I said, "but I'll bet you a ten-dollar hat that the test will come back that it's acid, low in organic matter, and poor in nitrogen, phosphate, and potash, and they'll recommend two tons of lime and 500 pounds of 5-10-5 mixed commercial fertilizer."

He laughed again. He also declined to take my bet. He'd seen too many tests come back like that before. He knew what the results would be.

But I went ahead and had the soil tests made. It came back just as we both had known it would. And here I parted company with the county agent and his system. I had vowed to forsake the chemical way of farming forever. I was determined to follow the organic method from then on. So, instead of putting on two tons of lime, as advised, we put on a half-ton of lime, 500 pounds of raw rock phosphate, and 500 pounds of raw rock potash. Then we planted the field in crimson clover.

I had no cattle on this field at this time. I just let the grass grow and let the clover grow. The first year we had a fair growth. In late summer we mowed the field and left the hay lying on the ground. I didn't make an attempt to bale it. I had had no intention of baling it.

By now the other farmers were making fun of us and our "unscientific" organic farming. "The good doctor's lost his mind. He's fooled around and lost his hay!" they chortled to each other.

We didn't lose the hay. It went exactly where we wanted it to go, right back into the good earth where it would increase the organic content and feed the earthworms and all the soil microorganisms that we knew were necessary to grow good crops.

So the first year we cut the hay and left it on the ground to nourish the soil. But from that point on this ground—and the other fields that I subsequently converted to the organic method—consistently grew better crops throughout the years. To accomplish this, we did two things: we didn't overgraze the field, and we didn't poison the land with commercial fertilizers. On the positive side, we fertilized with natural fertilizers, and we plowed the organic matter back in. Since that year this field has been used as a pasture. I planted Bahia seed, so that now we have a mixture of Bahia and bermuda grass in the summer and crimson clover in the winter. The clover puts good God-given free nitrogen into the soil through little nodules on the roots, which I am convinced is infinitely more valuable than the synthetic nitrogen that comes as nitrate in the NKP fertilizers. It also adds to the organic content with its deep roots that delve down to bring up various minerals from the earth. This process, a relatively easy one and also relatively inexpensive, also broke up the hardpan that was a characteristic of this worn-out farm that had been mined for generations. There's no more hardpan; there's life in the soil. Today it's growing healthy cattle.

That's how I changed one pasture.

I have given you the story of just one field, to demonstrate on a small scale what can be done. The principles vary little from state to state, from small to large-scale farming. What happened in my one little field also happened on a larger scale in all of Cass County, where I live, when we set out in another way to restore the health of our soil. And it has happened on farm after farm in Iowa and many other states. I can speak from the knowledge of personal experience and first-hand observation when I tell you of my corner of Texas and of large-scale farming operations in Iowa's corn belt. I've seen those changes and had a hand in them, and they worked fine. I think the people found the only satisfactory solution there was.

Here, first, is what happened close to home, not on my farm but in my home county.

When I came to Atlanta, Texas, in 1933 the land was exhausted. Farmers had planted corn one year and cotton the next, just as had been done on my own 1,000-acre farm. The pattern continued with boring regularity; always taking out. They were using commercial fertilizers in an increasing tempo. Soon the rolling hills that are a characteristic of our homeland had lost their fertility. Much of the topsoil had washed into the Red River and from it into the Mississippi and thence into the Gulf of Mexico.

World War II came. Renewing their determination to grow more food and fiber for the war effort, the citizen-farmers went all out. They doused the land with commercial fertilizer, to produce more food. Nor was this enough. During the war, *fifty-seven* peckerwood sawmills came into the little county and indiscriminately chewed up the timber for lumber. A peckerwood sawmill is a small operation that just sets up and starts sawing away at whatever's in sight. By the time the war was over, they had cut down nearly every tree that would make a two-by-four.

By 1945 disaster hung over the county. The land was almost completely ruined, ravaged of its trees, the soil depleted. The farmers could no longer make a living on the land. They moved to town. Cass County had lost one-fourth of its population. It was a critical moment in the area's history.

In that year of disaster, 1945, the Marion-Cass Soil Conservation District was organized and I became one of its directors. We were aware of the county's critical condition and in that first year we set out to accomplish only one goal. We set out to plant pine trees, in this way to restore the fertility of our soil. We were trying to use each acre of land for the purpose it was suited for; most of the acreage in these rolling hills was ideally suited for pines. Pines gave the land a rest from its overcultivation and overcutting. Over a period of a few years we planted forty million pine trees. As a result of this, a large paper company is building a $72 million plant to utilize this valuable natural resource.

But we did not lose our sense of balance and plant the whole wide country in pine trees. After we had our tree-planting program well established, we initiated a campaign to improve pastures and grasslands. We adopted a slogan, "Turn the District Green." Just as we had encouraged pine-tree planting, now we urged farmers to plant Austrian winter peas, vetch, and crimson clover, all legumes that would put free nitrogen back into the soil along with organic matter.

We also began to make use of two fine local agricultural industries we have—chickens and cattle. When a chicken industry came to town we told our farmers to utilize the chicken litter on the land as a fertilizer that would restore the fertility. They did so. This led to the growth of a very prosperous cattle industry in our county—and more animal manures. In time we restored the fertility to thousands and thousands of acres. This campaign resulted in our winning first prize in state competition as the best soil conservation district in Texas. The district gained $1,000 in prize money.

We were not content to stop there either. Several years later we began another campaign, this time to grow gardens. We made a slogan, "Let's Everybody Plant a Garden," and gave prizes for the best gardens, hoping to encourage everyone to have fresh natural, poison-free food grown on fertile soil. We gave extra points if the gardener had a compost pile. As people begin to recognize the better all-around qualities, and the superior taste, of these home-grown, poison-free vegetables, the idea is spreading more and more.

More recently, we started an anti-pollution campaign. We gained the backing of the county judge and the county commissioners, and went into the rural communities of the county and dug pits in the ground where we buried trash that the city people from other counties were bringing in and dumping on us. The citizens responded with enthusiasm. They wanted to have a clean county. The program became a very popular one; requests to explain it came from civic clubs such as Rotary. Using "before-and-after" types of colored slides to demonstrate our effectiveness, I began making speeches to all the interested organizations. Out of this came the invitation to make the speech to the state meeting of the Texas State Soil Conservation Districts. The topic apparently held some appeal there, for next I was invited to make the speech at a regional meeting at Hot Springs, Arkansas, where soil conservationists from the states of Arkansas, Oklahoma, Louisiana, and Texas had gathered.

As it turned out, these were steps up the ladder to the national convention of Soil and Water Conservation Districts, which met in Atlanta, Georgia, in 1969, where I was invited to make the same anti-pollution speech. There were three speakers on the program that morning, and each of us was allotted twenty minutes. But luckily for me the first two speakers (I was last) used only ten minutes each. That left me a bountiful forty minutes and I was determined to pack as much as I could into those forty minutes. Ted Elders, a member of our soil conservation district who accompanied me to the national convention, and I worked out a system for cramming in all the points we could. Ted would roll the color slides into the projector while, as quickly and as efficiently as I could, I would present the anti-pollution speech that I had delivered at the previous state and regional conferences.

My regular program completed, then I told that group of leaders and good farmers and men in various aspects of agriculture that I thought I knew how to stop the city people from dumping all these tin cans and bottles all over our land. If something weren't done to stop it soon, I told them, we were going to be knee deep in cans and loose paper.

Immediately one man called out, "What can we do?"

"Here's what we can do," I said. "Let's go to the city people and make a promise. Tell them if they'll stop dumping all this rubbish on us, we'll stop putting poison in their foods: we'll stop spraying DDT and cancer-causing chemicals all over the fruits and vegetables they have to eat!"

It was a timely topic at that agricultural convention. Ever since publication of Rachel Carson's *Silent Spring* the problem of pesticides has been an area of growing concern in America. These men in Atlanta, Georgia, that day realized something had to be done soon. It had begun to concern them intimately. Everywhere I subsequently went on that convention floor, small groups motioned me in to discuss this whole problem of agricultural chemicals.

We are living in changing times. The main reason change is urgently needed and is occurring in agriculture is that chemical farming is in crisis. Not only is chemical agriculture making the nation and its farmers both sick, it is becoming more and more expensive each year. Of course, there are increased equipment and labor costs, but the primary precipitant of this crisis is the escalation of chemical treatment of the crops with both synthetic fertilizers and poisons. The crisis hurts both economically and medically. Farmers are in a great dilemma. They want to get out of their trap. They certainly don't want to poison this nation, nor themselves. They are seeking timely changes for these changing times, and many of them are changing their whole philosophies toward farming. They are changing over to the organic method, and they are making money, and they are regaining their health.

It is encouraging to see these changes come, for it was not this way at all in the very early history of Natural Food Associates. In those days Tom Lavin and I traveled all over this country, flying in DC-3s at night to save money, trying to spread the NFA story, and people weren't much interested in what we were talking about. It was difficult for us to get together a very big audience.

One night many years ago Tom and I flew to Omaha, Nebraska. At Omaha we rented a car and drove on to Fremont, Nebraska. Nine persons showed up for the meeting. This great turnout probably would have discouraged some people, but the trip became worthwhile for me because those nine were interested. They took the trouble to go out that night and listen to us. The fact that many such groups were small back in the 1950s did not deter us. As far as I am concerned, that was pioneering work, and pioneers must learn not to expect great results overnight. It has taken those years to bring the people of this country, ever so slowly, to realize the dangers we all face today.

One of our fellow pioneers we acquired almost by accident. Dr. Lloyd Church, a dentist, had helped solve the water problem in Oklahoma. He had joined NFA, and I asked him to be on our program. When it came time for his speech, he requested that his time be split with a friend of his, Joseph A. Cocannouer. I took one good look at his friend and I became anxious. Cocannouer wore a string tie and a wool shirt, his suit was unpressed; he looked like another "whang-brain" to me, a real old hayseed. I explained to Dr. Church that we had a rule in NFA against unscheduled speakers.

But Dr. Church, sensing my first impression of his friend, said, "He'll make a better speech than I, and probably better than you, Dr. Joe."

So we broke the rule and let Cocannouer speak. He was a great success. We all enjoyed it. I'm not even sure today what he spoke on. It was probably of weeds or nature in general. This author-professor-scientist had a personality that came through.

I came to share many a speaker's table with Cocannouer. He had a color all his own. His hair usually needed combing, and we finally made him buy a new suit of clothes, but once he started talking—or writing—he enjoyed instant communication.

He was an expert on soil science and conservation. He was the former head of soils and horticulture at the College of Tropical Agriculture in The Philippines and had taught in several other colleges and universities. He had broadcast agricultural information over the Voice of America. And out of his long life he had a wealthy storehouse of fascinating experiences to draw from. In many ways he was an apt symbol of timely changes for changing times.

When he became active in NFA, Cocannouer had never flown before in his life. He used buses and trains solely for travel. He was urged to make this timely change for these changing times. Surface travel just took too long for the traveling we had to do.

"You're going to have to fly," I told him.

Finally he capitulated. "If you and Lavin'll meet me in Tulsa, I'll fly from Tulsa to Minnesota," where we were going that weekend, he promised.

We got on a DC-6. Once he was on the plane, up high, he looked out the window and got on Cloud Nine from being able to see everything. Soon he began regaling all of us around him, fellow passengers and stewardess, with stories of his years of teaching agriculture in The Philippines. He was sent to an island. He knew how to get along with people, and he was a scientist—a botanist. He was a naturalist who could go into the jungle and know which berry or plant he could safely eat. Thus he quickly became popular with the natives. The chief of the tribe adopted him as a son. But this meant he automatically got twelve wives. How was he to select them? Well, Cocannouer knew how to get along with people. There were three age groups in that tribe. He took four brides out of each group. Balance.

That trip to Minnesota was the fastest most of us had ever taken. Cocannouer's death a few years ago was more than a personal loss to those of us in NFA; it was a loss to the country.

We're still traveling all over America, and today it is easy to see that times have changed. Instead of tiny clots of people, such as we found to greet us that night in Fremont, we find packed meeting places with hundreds of people, and they are all deeply interested. They are sick, they know they're sick, and they're coming in droves to try to find some answers.

One of the best examples I know with which to demonstrate the temper of these changing times and to illustrate how chemical farming can be replaced with organic methods is what I have seen in Iowa's great Corn Belt. In 1964, a group of farmers invited me to go to Cedar Rapids, Iowa, and talk to them about the nitrate problem. The deep, dark land in Iowa is some of the world's most fertile soil. But since the early 1950s most farmers in Iowa had been using excessive amounts of synthetic nitrogen fertilizers as they planted corn on the same ground year after year. Their wells were "hot" from the nitrates that had seeped from their fields into the underground water supply and thence into their drinking water. They were losing money. Their cattle were not reproducing properly and were not gaining weight as they should have been. The year before, they had had a drouth and when they had cut up some strains of corn for silage, the corn blew up the silos, and the juice that ran out of the silos killed the cows, ducks, chickens, or pigs that drank it. They carried the animals and corn samples to the agricultural experiment station at Ames, Iowa, and discovered the answer. Their problem was diagnosed as nitrate poisoning. The corn was so heavily fertilized with synthetic nitrogen that it was producing a feed that was deficient in vitamins A, E, and D. In the presence of excessive nitrates, the corn plant is unable to convert carotene (pro-vitamin A) into vitamin A. The answer the farmers were given at Ames was to inject vitamins A, D, and E into their animals. This did temporarily relieve the symptoms, but it had not solved the problem.

It was with this background, in the midst of a deep crisis, that 500 farmers came out to hear me in Cedar Rapids, Iowa, that night. They recognized their crisis. They knew it was close to a life-or-death situation. They were ripe for change as I told them the NFA story and what to do about their nitrate problem, how to grow good foods that were not poisoned, and how to restore and maintain the fertility of their soils.

These farmers, who owned some of the best land in America's heartland, were having huge veterinarian bills; some were actually going broke. One man told me he was spending $78 an acre on agricultural chemicals—fertilizer, weedicides, and pesticides; yet, although he was still making a high production in terms of bushels, he was losing money every year. Obviously he could not go on that way. He was fast reaching the point of financial asphyxiation.

This man, Francis Winkowitsch, changed over completely from chemical to organic farming. I suggested to him that if he wanted to solve the nitrate problem he first should stop using the synthetic nitrogen. Instead of planting corn on the same acreage every year, he should rotate his crops, a recognized practice that all good farmers followed. Going to full annual rotation, he should plant in a site corn one year, soybeans the next, followed in turn by oats, alfalfa, clover, or similar crops. And in other ways he should work organic matter back into the soil Then I told him, and his fellow farmers there that night, to get rid of the turning plow, or moldboard plow, which was the enemy of the farmer. The farmers who had settled the land back in the nineteenth century had found a tough sod; in order to break it, they used a deep plow to turn it way under so they could plant. But the moldboard or turning plow turns over the organic matter of the topsoil and buries it underneath the ground where it can't live. It brings clay to the top and ruins the living conditions of the soil micro-organisms. This destroys the topsoil, which is the life of the land. To replace the turning plow, I advised them to use the chisel plow, which would break up the hardpan that they all had by then and would aerate the soil as necessary for proper growth of their crops.

Essentially, what I told them that night boiled down to four steps or rules: stop using synthetic nitrates; rotate crops; replace the turning plow with the chisel plow, and instead of grazing off the organic matter, they should leave it on the ground and work it back into the soil by disking it into the topsoil.

Five years later Francis Winkowitsch had eliminated disease on his farm in both his plants and animals, was making a good profit, and was farming for himself instead of for the chemical people. His veterinarian bill dropped dramatically to a negligible annual figure. Each year his bank account was increasing.

What better proof can a man have of the superiority of the organic method?

One farmer summed it up, pointing at the earthworm castings on his farm: "That's my fertilizer now."

Restoring soil fertility and eliminating the harmful insects are two major steps toward successful farming that are tied together. The most effective way in which to eliminate the damage of insects is through biological control. But if a farmer has balance on his organic farm, he has biological control as a beneficial side effect. Alternating his crops contributes to balance and aids in pest control without dangerous poisons. Variety of growing plants, rather than an unbroken pattern of sameness, helps prevent disease. But acres and acres of the same crop attracts hordes of insects. When crops are not rotated annually, the problem is intensified.

When we have attained a balance of nature, we have a biological control of insects. This means we do not destroy the useful insects. One reason we have so great a problem in many locales is that the useful insects have been destroyed by mass spraying techniques. The ladybug is one of the farmer's best friends. In many places, small farmers have brought in ladybugs and praying mantes to help provide this biological control. Until this balance is achieved, of course, we will still have to use the old-time insecticides, in many instances. Rotenone, pyrethrum, ryania, and sabadilla dust were used before World War II successfully; they come from plants, are degradable, and do not cause cancer.

Balance is the key throughout. Green matter has to be completely decomposed before it is used and the land is planted. Never turn it *under*. Instead, disk it *in*. Disk in the top two or three inches of soil. To restore fertility, we need to observe closely what nature does and then seek to follow that blueprint. This means we should never cut in a green cover crop and plant right behind it. If we do, the bugs will probably eat up the crop. When we cut in cover crops like Austrian winter peas or vetch, we have to wait six weeks before planting. This gives the disked-in cover crop time to decompose. Decomposition takes time. Nature never does anything in a hurry. Man is more impatient than nature, but to get the results that nature does in enriching the soil, man must learn to operate on a schedule that allows for a more gradual decomposition. If he rushes the schedule, such as planting immediately after plowing in his green matter, then he is doing what the boy does when he eats a green apple. The boy couldn't wait for the apple to get ripe. But eating green apples is not nature's way. As a result, the boy gets a bellyache. The same thing happens, roughly, when nature's way is hurried by planting on top of the cover crop. The soil, to stretch an analogy to the bursting point, gets a bellyache.

Nature's way, in the long run, is the most profitable example to follow. This policy extends even into the type of seed a person buys for his farm or garden. Let's examine corn that is grown in this country.

Fungus disease has been known in corn for many years in the South, but suddenly in 1970 it began spreading northward to areas where it had never been before. In the worst places, as much as 90 per cent of the corn crop had been destroyed. Estimates of damage over the entire nation varied. The truth is unknown, but some put the figures at 10 to 15 per cent. It was, for instance, serious in Illinois, but less serious in Iowa. The disease gradually spread north into the corn-growing areas, in America's Corn Belt of the Middle West.

The price of corn immediately went up. In order to hold the prices down, the government began marketing the corn surplus that had been stored. But the crop remained short and the higher valuation of corn was reflected in the increased prices of chicken, beef, pork, and eggs.

To me the corn market headache traced back to a new type of corn seed that had been developed and was growing in popularity. It was a new hybrid variety developed by a geneticist in

Florida. He had bred a gene into the male plant that made it unnecessary to manually detassel the female plant. This was a development of considerable economic significance, for it saved seed growers worlds of money. It eliminated a step in preparation of corn seed, thereby cutting down on labor costs.

But, in my opinion, the corn grown from this seed had lost its resistance to disease, which accounted for the rapid spread of the corn fungus to areas where it had hitherto been practically unknown. A friend of mine who was an old, uneducated farmer didn't need a formal education to realize what had happened.

"The corn done lost its strength," he said. "Man been messing with Nature too much."

Stripped of jargon and scientific terminology and put into plain, simple everyday language, that was exactly what had happened.

Furthermore, hybrid corns do not contain the nutritional values that are found in open-pollinated varieties. There is even a Biblical injunction against hybrid seed in Leviticus, when the Lord told Moses, "thou shalt not sow thy field with mingled seed." For one thing, hybrid corn doesn't contain cobalt. That makes it a fragmented food, because corn ought to contain cobalt. Cobalt is necessary in human nutrition because it's a part of vitamin B_{12}. Nor does the quality of protein found in hybrid corn equal the protein of open-pollinated corn.

I have a friend who is a vocational agriculture teacher. He plants hybrid corn and gets a large yield every year. Then he sells the high-yield hybrid corn. He sells all of it. Doesn't he keep any for livestock feed? No, he doesn't. He *buys* open-pollinated corn to feed his cows and horses. Why? Well, he says they just do better on the open-pollinated variety.

The sale of open-pollinated corn seed is increasing in America today. Farmers realize they can grow adequate amounts with it. It is a part of organic corn-growing: a good quality corn in abundance without using chemical fertilizer and hybrid seed.

The lure of higher-yield hybrid seed has been exhibited to me, too. One year I had a beautiful corn crop on my own Jonica Farm. There were big stalks and ears, with dark green big leaves. I was going to make 75 to 100 bushels an acre, but the county agent told me if I had used hybrid seed and commercial fertilizer I could have expected to make 150 to 200 bushels an acre—twice as much. I agreed with him that I could have, but I pointed out that, at the same time, I would have been destroying my land and I would have been growing corn of inferior quality. In time I would have had the same thing at Jonica Farm that a few years later was happening in Iowa, nitrate poisoning and sickness in my animals. Corn of inferior quality, I am convinced, leads to sickness.

The open-pollinated corn is that of the oldtime varieties with its silk, or tassel, streaming out at the end of the ear. It pollinates itself so that you know what to expect from each year's seed. It reproduces itself in a dependable pattern, so that you can use your own seed with confidence each year. But hybrid corn will not reproduce itself with reliability. It will sprout and grow, but it won't grow true to form. You may get a little nubbin—or nothing. In addition, who knows the keeping quality of this hybrid corn from a patch touched by blight—or how much it will take to properly raise a hog? There are many economic factors to be considered here other than the one of mere quantity. The simple fact that the farmer has to buy new seed corn every year increases the financial burden of farming. Thus, the use of hybrid seed corn ties the farmer to the seed dealer; he can't risk growing his own. As in the marketing of degerminated wheat and infertile eggs, there is a large economic motive behind the use of hybrid corn, and the motive is not the farmer's.

But there is a choice for the farmer who knows the difference. He can still buy either kind of seed he wants. All the big seed companies produce open-pollinated seed corn also, and the farmer can buy open-pollinated corn from the same companies where he can buy the hybrid variety.

In changing over from the chemical to the organic method of farming, selection of seed is but one aspect, and at first, of course, it is secondary to the changes that must be made in the soil. Organic fertilizers and minerals are necessary for organic farming. When the big farmer, with several hundred or thousands of acres, changes over to organic methods he will need additional organic fertilizers. Today his problem is not as acute as once it would have been. Organic fertilizer can now be bought in a sack or packaged just like ordinary commercial fertilizer. There are deposits of raw rock phosphate and potash, marine trace minerals, and other deposits.

It has been found that after a few years of applying these organic rock fertilizers it is no longer necessary to use them. This is the vast difference in the two competing methods. The chemical farmer has to put on more and more every year. Chemical fertilizing becomes an expensive habit. But the organic farmer puts on less and less every year. This means that in the future the organic farmer is the one who will make the money, because it's not costing him as much to operate.

The farmer with extensive acreage invariably argues that he can't find enough organic matter for his farm. He has come to believe this because he has been told he must steal from one acre to get natural fertilizer for another acre. This is not true. He can get raw rock fertilizer at a cost not greater than regular commercial fertilizer would cost him. But where? he always asks. Actually, some feed stores stock it. It takes only a few phone calls to find out whether the local ones sell it or not. I always tell people, "Join NFA and look in the yellow pages of our monthly magazine." However you approach it, sources of supply are abundant. In every area of the country there are dealers who sell raw rock fertilizers or marine deposits. The big—or little—farmer just doesn't have to steal organic matter from one acre to get it in another acre. If he doesn't buy it, he can grow his own organic matter on every acre. He can do it himself by adhering to a few simple rules: don't "burn" by overgrazing; don't use chemicals; plow the organic matter in; plant deep-rooted plants; rotate the crops.

I have said it before in this book, but it is worth reminding that a fertile soil is a soil in which the conditions are optimum for the growth of soil micro-organisms. A fertile soil is a living soil. In order to make the optimum conditions, the Ph, or acid-alkaline balance, must be near the neutral point. If the Ph is too high, there is an alkaline condition. If it's too low, the soil is too acid. If either extreme exists, then the trace minerals are locked up and the conditions are not optimum. The effect on the farmer's results tends to be the same, although there are some plants and flowers that do well in a slightly acid soil.

Balance is the secret, whether it is in farming or in nutrition. Some soils may even become high in organic matter and not grow good crops. This is true in muck soils, for instance. But when there is balance, there is a Ph balance, there is organic matter, there is aeration, and the soil has a water-holding capacity. Soil micro-organisms must have air; thus it is tremendously important to break up the hardpan and allow air into the soil. Aeration further promotes the growth of soil micro-organisms. The soil needs water, and organic matter helps hold in the water. By using a chisel plow on hardpan land, the water sinks into the soil instead of washing off the top. We might say it percolates instead of floods. Organic matter soaks up water like a sponge; this helps the soil to maintain a proper moisture level.

The restoration of the soil's fertility, in my opinion, would go a long way toward solving problems of floods and water shortages, which will never be solved until we restore the organic matter to the soil. The usual 100 pounds of soil in my own county won't hold 30 pounds of water, but 100 pounds of humus holds 195 pounds of water like a sponge. In a society in which the shortage of water is already recognized as one of the future's critical problems, this fact is a crucial one. The construction of dams on rivers will never completely solve the water problem. A dam only treats the symptoms of the disease. The underground water level in this country will continue to fall until we restore organic matter to the soil. We must learn how to trap the raindrop where it falls, instead of washing our topsoil into the rivers.

Can the organic method be applied to all kinds of agriculture? I see no reason why not. A point in case is the cotton farmer. The cotton farmer has been told—and he believes it—that he cannot grow cotton the organic way. But many of them have found that they can't grow it the chemical way anymore either, because they are fast going bankrupt. The use of synthetic fertilizers and insecticides makes the overhead almost prohibitive. Without the government subsidy now, all of them would go broke. They couldn't produce cotton that could compete in the world market. It seems more logical to say that the government is subsidizing the chemical industry, not the farmer. The chemical industry is getting more cotton money than is the farmer.

I have some friends who grow cotton the organic way. They restore fertility of their soils with legumes and raw rock fertilizers. And they still have some insect problems, but they use diatomaceous earth, containing silica from small fossils, to control these insects. Diatomaceous earth, very popular today and being used in quantity, is a marine deposit that has been ground up into very fine particles. It destroys the insect after contact by mechanical means by simply piercing its skin and the insect "bleeds" to death. It is very satisfactory on various insects and worms, and very well suited for all kinds of gardening and farming as well as cotton culture. It is non-toxic and can be used as a mineral supplement for livestock. Pyrethrum can be added for use by the organic farmer to control cabbage worms and other garden insects.

One of the chief reasons why it is hard for the cotton farmer to switch to the organic method is that cotton heretofore has suffered from such vast applications of modern insecticides that practically all of the beneficial insects have been destroyed. It takes time for the beneficial insects to return. What makes it worse, the damaging insects such as the boll worm and the boll weevil are frequently found to be immune to DDT. When one pesticide no longer controls the insects, the farmer is forced to resort to other powerful insecticides. At present, cotton farmers are using toxaphene and even parathion, one of the most deadly insecticides known to man.

The cost of chemical farming is so high that were it not for bountiful government subsidies, cotton farmers would be jumping out of windows all the way from Memphis to New Orleans, until they clogged the Mississippi River. That is, they would clog the Mississippi unless they began working their way out of this chemical farming maze. The best way to start would be to take their land out of cotton and put it back into grass. Grass is the great healer. Planting grass and letting it grow is the way to restore the fertility of the soil. It also brings back the useful insects. Many cotton farmers have already found it necessary to do this.

Some farmers will tell you that vegetables, as well as cotton, cannot be grown without the use of modern insecticides. But how did we do it before World War II, before the days of our modern insecticides? Prior to 1946, the year that DDT entered the agricultural market, America's farmers did grow crops without such extremely poisonous, highly persistant chemical poisons. Other such dangerous compounds followed DDT on the market. But were they necessary? Well, when I was a boy we grew perfectly good vegetables and fruits without using any of the modern insecticides. Our trees had host resistance to disease. If we grew vegetables and fruits before World War II without the high-risk, often cancer-causing pesticides that are so common today, then we can do the same job today in the same way. But everywhere I go I am asked this question:

"Well, Doctor, how do you control insects?"

On our own Jonica Farm, the first thing we did to control insects was to restore the fertility of the soil. A fertile soil grows a healthy plant that does not attract insects. The bugs and worms tend to gravitate toward a plant, or a field of plants, that has already been weakened by disease or improper development. But this often is not sufficient, so that some use of insecticides may be required. This does not mean we should give up and go buy the powerful pesticides that are so highly advertised, because there *are* certain insecticides that are perfectly permissible to use. These are the oldtime pesticides that are made from plants, such as rotenone and pyrethrum. Since they come from plants themselves, they are rapidly degradable and are not cancer-causing. They do the job, and they are safe, and they are inexpensive. What more could we ask of an insecticide?

For the farmer with large acreage, as much as 500 or 1,000 acres, it may not be practical to change over to the organic way all in one year, as did the Iowa farmer we mentioned earlier in this chapter. What worked for him may not spell success for another, for varying reasons. Furthermore, most people wouldn't want to change over so rapidly. For those owning a large farm who would like to convert to the organic method gradually, it would be profitable to start off with 40 acres at first. He would change that 40 acres completely the first year. He would use no chemicals on that piece of land and he would build up the fertility with organic matter. But he would farm the rest of his land as he had been doing for years.

The chances are that those 40 acres, even in the first year, would tell him much about the two different methods. The following year he could make perhaps half of his farm organic. Convinced by these pilot programs, he could have a completely organic farm in his third year. In this way we would have changed over one step at a time, which would give him time to see the results first before going all-out. This is a practical approach, starting with 40 acres or a portion of a farm, and then enlarging the organic portion each year. Many large farmers do it this way; it's ideally suited for a cautious, practical man.

The organic way is even more important in regions of the South and on sandy soils. In the South where it's hot the farmer with poor land simply compounds his problem when he uses commercial fertilizer. Commercial fertilizer burns out the organic matter much quicker; the farmer goes broke that much quicker. Yet this has happened all over the South, on some of our most fertile soils. The blacklands north of Dallas, Texas, have been almost destroyed by the use of chemical fertilizers. As more and more chemicals have been used, cotton and corn production has steadily decreased, and the farmers have found they have to replace the organic matter in the soils.

In sandy soils, commercial fertilizer leaches out and goes downstream into rivers and lakes where it encourages growth of algae and weeds of all kinds. It enters underground water also, further compounding the pollution problem. Eventually it leads to putrification of the lakes. Too much organic matter burns up the oxygen of the water. Lake Erie is a prime example of a dead lake in America today. This huge lake has been killed. Most people blame its death on the sewage that has gone into the lake. Sometimes they mention commercial fertilizer. The fact is that the extensive use of commercial fertilizer around Lake Erie is a major cause of its putrification. And, what makes it worse, the farmer hasn't had a return for his fertilizer money. It has washed away, polluting the world for others, too.

Many people wonder how the organic cotton farmer in the South can maintain the organic content of his soils. Certainly with a crop like cotton that greedily depletes the soil, he must take steps to *keep* his land fertile. Yet he doesn't have the problem that the chemical farmer has, because chemicals kill the earthworm, destroy soil bacteria, and burn out the organic material in the soil. In order to maintain the fertility of his soil, the cotton farmer must learn to plant more cover crops. Vetch and Austrian winter peas can be planted and disked back into the soil to recover organic matter before spring planting time. Rye and oats can also be used for winter grazing; this is a very practical method. Another thing the cotton farmer must incorporate into his overall plan is the annual rotation of crops. He can't continue to plant the same crop on the same piece of land year after year. He may plant cotton one year, soybeans the next or, in some places, alfalfa. This is the same lesson the Midwestern corn farmer has learned. On the plains of Texas, they have learned to rotate cotton and soybeans, and they disk the stubble back into the ground where it belongs.

Proof of the pudding, they used to say, is in the eating. Today all over America farmers are changing over to the organic way. Hundreds of farmers are growing corn in Iowa by organic methods. Other farmers, large and small, are asking questions about organic farming. They are trying it, and liking it, and finding that it puts money into their pockets. Times have changed. I think a new day is dawning.

XIII.

Scientific Suicide

"Never be the first to take up the new, nor the last to discard the old."

I first heard that statement decades ago from a professor of mine at the University of Arkansas Medical School. It made a deep and lasting impression on me. Today, in my sixties, I believe more than ever that it is a valid guide especially in the practice of medicine. If we as a nation had followed this guide in our practice of agriculture, we would not be in nearly as much trouble as we are today.

Instead of following this precept, we in this country have been following a path I call "scientific suicide," for we have allowed chemical experimentation upon our people in the guise of "science." I do not mean that it is science applied in what I consider the true spirit of science, free of economic motivation. Economic motivation is often behind this scientific suicide. In many instances, scientists thinking only of the public good are caught up in the process without realizing it. There are many aspects to it. Chemical experimentation or chemical exploitation for economic gain—whatever the terminology adopted, we must halt it everywhere in this country, if we are to regain our national health. We must take a new, clearer, harder look at that which we have been calling "science." Is it scientific or not? Are we headed toward a scientific suicide?

The late Dr. Tom Douglas Spies, regarded as an authority in the field of nutrition, summed it up when he accepted the Distinguished Service Award from the American Medical Association a few years ago. "All diseases are caused by chemicals," he said, "and all diseases can be cured by chemicals. All the chemicals used by the body—except for the oxygen which we breathe and the water which we drink—are taken in through food. If we only knew enough, all diseases could be prevented, and could be cured, through proper nutrition. As tissues become damaged because they lack the chemicals of good nutrition, they tend to become old. They lack what I call 'tissue integrity.' There are people of 40 whose brains and arteries are senile. If we can help the tissues repair themselves by correcting nutritional deficiencies, we can make old age wait."

This is what I call a responsible statement, one that, accepted in all its implications, could slow down our trend toward scientific suicide.

What are examples of the diseases caused by chemicals? They are legend. Let us begin with our old enemy, hydrogenated fats. The consumption of hydrogenated fats continues to increase, despite definite, scientifically-demonstrated evidence that these fats are the chief villain in causing heart disease. Of course, the producers of edible fats have their own answer to this, because their profits are being threatened. With hundreds of thousands of dollars, perhaps even more, dedicated to publicity efforts, they claim that "fats have not been proven guilty." This is a process of public obfuscation. Fats *have* been proved guilty. Dr. L. W. Kinsell of Oakland, California, in a careful three-year study, placed the chief blame for atherosclerosis upon hydrogenated fats. He also proved that natural oils, high in the essential fatty acids, will consistently lower the cholesterol level and aid in the treatment of cardiovascular disease. Low fat diets, once commonly prescribed, do not necessarily lower blood cholesterol in atherosclerotic individuals, and as a matter of fact Dr. Kinsell placed his patients on a very high fat diet. But he gave them *natural* oils that are high in the essential unsaturated fatty acids.

Arachidonic acid is regarded as the primary essential fatty acid. It occurs only in insignificant amounts in the average daily dietary. Linoleic acid, another essential fatty acid, requires vitamin B_6 for its conversion into arachidonic acid. Thus the body depends on the dietary intake of both linoleic acid and vitamin

B_6 for normal cholesterol levels. This means that the prevention of cardiovascular disease depends upon not only an adequate intake of natural oils but vitamin B_6 as well. Choline, another part of the vitamin B complex, has been proved to be necessary for proper fat metabolism. But the addition of synthetic vitamin B_6 alone with natural oils is not the proper approach. Adequate intake of natural vitamin B that contains all of the factors both known and unknown is the sensible and logical approach. Our national dietary is also deficient in this natural vitamin B complex, chiefly because of the robbery that occurs in the processing and cooking of our foods.

Studies have also shown that a high refined carbohydrate intake can produce a marked hypercholesterolemia and that the greater the intake of refined carbohydrate, the greater the requirement for unsaturated fatty acids. Thus the consumption of white sugar and synthetic glucose, generally accepted as a chief cause of dental caries, now is exposed as a factor in our increasing cardiovascular disease. In their search for the cause of heart disease, some of our best researchers have also stumbled upon the truth about concentrated, fragmented sweets.

The medical director of one of our largest insurance companies has told me that cardiovascular diseases account for 64 per cent of his death claims. I doubt that this figure will change much until the American people come to realize the dangers of hydrogenated fats and white sugar and glucose.

It is for these reasons that I no longer use the diets recommended by the American Diabetes Association. The diets include foods that I consider junk foods, which cause diabetes and heart disease. Although physicians accepted as authorities in the field of diabetes recommend such diets, I must respectfully disagree with them. Furthermore, I am convinced that diabetes can be controlled by diet. I explain to my patients, at great length, that diabetes is a metabolic disease that involves not only carbohydrate metabolism but also the metabolism of fats and proteins. They must not only avoid all refined carbohydrates but also hydrogenated fats and proteins of poor quality. They must avoid all white flour products, including white biscuits and commercial spaghetti and macaroni and noodles. They must not eat soda crackers since the soda cracker is made from white flour, shortening, refined salt, and soda. They are told to avoid commercial ice cream and peanut butter. These latter items are all included in current, widely-distributed diets for diabetes.

I tell the diabetic to use unrefined salt, natural cold-pressed oils, whole grain cereals, and honey that has not been pasteurized. Even a diabetic can eat small quantities of natural honey. The diabetic can eat all types of fresh fruits and vegetables. Nuts and seeds in moderation are encouraged. Whole grain breads from freshly ground organically grown wheat is directed. They may have baked Irish potatoes, but never creamed potatoes or potato chips.

About fifteen years ago, I had a patient with all of the classical symptoms of *diabetes mellitus*. He had lost 30 pounds and was underweight. I was his family doctor, but he had never been sick before. I had delivered his children and had been called when they were ill with the usual childhood diseases. He came into my office with all the symptoms of acute diabetes. His urine showed 4-plus sugar. His fasting blood sugar was 435 mg. per cent.

I scolded him for not coming in for an examination earlier. He already knew the diagnosis. He explained that his mother had been a diabetic and had required insulin shots during the last years of her life. He very frankly told me that he was not going to take insulin shots. If I insisted on giving him the shots he would find another doctor. I made him a counter offer. I made him agree that he would avoid all the junk foods on my list and eat only the foods that I recommended. I did not make him measure these foods because he was already underweight. I also made him promise to grow an organic garden.

He kept his promise. His strength returned, his blood pressure came down, he regained his normal weight, and his blood sugar came down to near normal limits.

He was an acute diabetic of the adult type, whose symptoms were controlled by proper nutrition. Of course, this man still has diabetes. Proper nutrition has at least prolonged his life. I suspect he has "sinned a little." He, like countless others, will cheat a little and eat "convenient junk foods." The relentless cardiovascular disease that plagues the diabetic will probably make his death certificate eventually read either coronary heart disease or stroke.

It is true that heredity was a factor in the cause of his diabetes. But years of malnutrition caused by his daily diet of refined salt, hydrogenated fats, white flour products, white sugar and glucose, and the dry cereals also played an important role in his disease. I am convinced that any diabetic, despite his inherited background, can prolong his life if he gets proper nutrition. I also believe that most symptomatic adult onset diabetes can be controlled by diet alone. I do not believe that oral hypoglycemic drugs are necessary.

When will our scientists learn that the answer to our nutritional problems is simply natural food grown on fertile soil? Or is it that the answer is too simple? Or is it that there are, too often, gigantic, strongly-motivated economic blocks in the way of finding that simple answer? When we have research grants of large sums going to our great universities and laboratories, we are justified in allowing our suspicions to grow at the results that come out of the consequent research. Is a grant from the Sugar Information, Inc. going to finance indictment of the sugar industry for dental caries? No one expects such a thing, and it will not happen. Research on health and nutrition must be clean money. It must be freely given with no thought of getting anything back except the truth about proper nutrition. This kind of money is hard to find.

There is at least a ray of hope on the horizon in cancer research. The Warburg theory is gaining the respect of many researchers. This theory holds that the cause of cancer is related to a derangement of the enzymatic processes in the cell. Literally thousands of enzymatic reactions are going on at all times in the individual cells, and anything that disturbs or disrupts these reactions may be a factor in causing cancer. We in NFA have been trying to show that natural food grown on fertile soil and poison free is perhaps the best way to obtain all of the essential amino acids, all the natural vitamins, and all the organic minerals. Enzymes are made from these nutrients, and it is reasonable to infer that a deficiency of any of them will cause a deranged enzymatic activity and a faulty metabolism. Of one thing we are certain: natural, poison-free food grown on fertile soil won't hurt anybody. I don't think our worst critics have ever claimed otherwise. If so, I haven't heard of it.

It is also known that many of the chemical additives in our foods are vitamin antagonists and enzyme inhibitors. Another group of chemicals that are proved to be enzyme inhibitors and vitamin antagonists are some of the drugs so commonly used today, the sulfas, the antibiotics, and many of the new "wonder" drugs. An increasing number of doctors are deploring their indiscriminate use. Millions of prescriptions are written annually for tranquilizers. Tranquilizers come in third, behind antibiotics and synthetic vitamins, in popularity.

I have been impressed by what I have read on "man-made disease." One article stated that "during the past 20 years, medical gains have produced several types of man-made disease." ACTH and cortisone are known to cause peptic ulcer. Vascular lesions in rheumatoid arthritis are often associated with steroid medication. Fungus infections, staphylococci enteritis, or vitamin deficiency may occur if the natural balance of gastro-intestinal organisms is upset by antibacterial agents. Prolonged use of oral antibiotics can be dangerous. Vitamin deficiencies are always more likely in undernourished patients. Antibiotics may reduce intestinal bacteria that normally produce vitamin K and several members of the vitamin B complex. Antihypertensive agents have various undesirable side effects. Many of them have been discarded because they were too dangerous. Liver disorders have been reported due to Thorazine, the popular tranquilizer. Each year, new items are added to the list.

There is, I fear, in the psychology of our people a dependency upon the "one-shot cure." Too many Americans yearn for a single treatment that will bring instant health. They seek the easy way that gives them what they want without having to change their style of life. This, in my opinion, is a dangerous tendency. I am reminded of our epidemics of Asian flu in this country. Millions of Americans have rolled up their sleeves and taken a hurriedly prepared vaccine to ward off a terrible new disease. But many of them got sick anyway, and the disease was not as terrible as it had been pictured. As a physician, this mass hysteria of our people to take unproved injections worries me. I hope nobody reports a case of African plague in this country.

Another danger that faces our country is the increasing use of chemical additives to our foods. Most of the chickens are fed arsenic and antibiotics. Cattle are often fed stilbestrol. Stilbestrol is known to induce cancer. Dr. Hanower, the father of endrocrinology in this country, has stated that "stilbestrol is a potent drug, and serious consequences may result unless it is used under constant medical supervision. Physicians who use this drug should be familiar with its indication, dosage, precautions, and particularly the possible detrimental effects. Extreme care should be taken to avoid overdosage. It is also desirable that the breasts and pelvic organics be examined before treatment is instituted as well as at frequent intervals during therapy." The dangers of continuous ingestion of this synthetic female sex hormone is described by Dr. Leonard Biskind, who concluded: "I cannot view this practice except with the gravest concern."*

Yet it is not easy to combat the trend toward the various forms of scientific suicide prevalent in our society. For one thing, it invites character assassination and ridicule. Dr. Edward J. Ryan, editor of the *Dental Digest,* summed it up perfectly. He said: "Anyone who speaks up against food adulteration in any of the many forms is subject to 'name calling.' The most common epithets are 'food faddist' or 'food fakir.' If you object to spraying foods with poisonous chemicals, picking fruits green and then applying a dye, to injecting or administering antibiotics to poultry and dairy herds, to removing minerals and vitamins from natural foods, to adding chemical adulterants to preserve foods from normal chemical changes, you are offending . . . some of our largest and most influential corporations. . . . We can be certain that the public relations counsellors will go to work to change the situation—even if that requires a bit of character assassination directed against those who are in the opposition. Every time that a natural substance is removed from a food, every time an adulterant is added to a food, the balance in nature is disturbed. . . . The chemical and cellular processes within the body cells cannot react to the passing whims of chemists without disturbance in function. It took thousands of years for the body to adjust itself to changing environmental conditions. When these conditions are suddenly altered by the actions of men, the cells cannot make the adjustment—disease is the result."

Although we have covered this ground before in this book, it is necessary to emphasize once again that the increasing use of chemical fertilizers and insecticides is another significant aspect of this scientific suicide I have been discussing. Not only do they produce inferior food, these chemicals are destroying the virgin natural fertility of our soils. Tests show that the organic content of our soils is decreasing everywhere these chemicals are used. They make land poor, instead of rich as they claim, and both the percentage and the quality of the protein diminish in poor soils. Yet high quality protein is essential to the survival of our nation.

**Modern Medicine,* Oct. 5, 1954.

These poor foods also contain poisons that in some cases are cancer-causing.

And the dangers of these poisons are apparent to many of those who are using them. A few years ago I happened to be in Arizona during the lettuce season. I looked up and saw a plane making a pass at a lettuce field. It left a trench of spray twenty feet wide and seven feet deep. They were spraying what I was told was parathion. Parathion is one of the deadliest poisons to humans.

"You eat that lettuce?" I asked a man there.

He grinned. "No, we send it to New York."

But that man was probably eating food that a farmer in another state had poisoned and sent to Arizona. In today's small world, the poison cycle eventually comes back to rest on one's own doorstep.

A few of our national leaders are beginning to see the dangers of this continued chemical onslaught upon our lands. But in most instances they seem powerless to stop it. Our agricultural colleges continue to graduate specialists who become vocational agricultural teachers in the schools and county agents who go forth to extol the virtues of poison insecticides, herbicides, and commercial fertilizers.

Some chemists, obviously, will not agree with what I say here. At a national soil conservation convention several years ago, I heard a soil scientist who is chairman of the department of soils at a large university tell the same sad story of our dilemma of increasing population and decreasing farm lands.

"We have nothing to fear," he said. "Farmers do not have to go to the trouble and expense of planting legumes. They can now buy all the nitrogen they need from 42 synthetic nitrogen factories who can make nitrogen from air." It sounded more like an advertisement for a chemical fertilizer company than careful, sound soil science. But how many others in positions like his say the same thing? The figures are likely to be depressing.

I am sure of this: synthetic nitrogen will not produce good quality food for a starving civilization. It will destroy the life of the soil. And somebody has got to save the soil; somebody has to restore its fertility, teach the farmer how to restore the fertility, how to restore the organic matter in our soils if our growing population is to be fed. Unless someone meets this challenge, famine, starvation, and disease will result. The U.S. Department of Agriculture and the state land grant colleges must face this issue because they are the responsible agents, but until now they have not met this responsibility. One of NFA's objectives is to teach them the vital facts about soil life, soil restoration, and soil conservation, for we are convinced that only organic farming methods will save our land and insure an adequate food supply for our children.

The historical American way of dealing with nature has been exploitative. In this country we talk of helping underprivileged countries whose standards of living are very low. Our leaders mention that these nations have neither the money nor the scientific know-how to "exploit their natural resources." Then the clincher invariably is that we must take the lead and show them the scientific way to "exploit" their natural resources. I have no doubt that we can demonstrate this to them. We have already done it in America. But will this exploitation of natural resources lead to peace in the world? I doubt it seriously. If our leaders continue to teach exploitation both here and abroad, war will inevitably result. When America becomes hungry enough as a result of exploiting our own natural resources, we will become a war-like nation ready to invade any foreign land where we can find food. This is a lesson of history. Japan went into Manchuria looking for protein from the soybean. Peace in this world is dependent upon the *conservation* of natural resources, not their *exploitation.*

W. C. Lowdermilk, formerly assistant chief of the Soil Conservation Service, made an 18-month tour of western Europe, North Africa, and the Middle East to study soil erosion and land use in those areas. He hoped to use the data gleaned there to help do something about the soil erosion problem in this country. In the process of reporting what he had learned, Lowdermilk also came up with some general observations that are as pertinent today as when he wrote them. He said:

"A just relation of peoples to the earth rests not on exploitation, but rather on conservation—not on the dissipation of resources, but rather on restoration of the productive powers of the land and on access to food and raw materials. If civilization is to avoid a long decline, like the one that has blighted North Africa and the Near East for 13 centuries, society must be born again out of an economy of *exploitation* into an economy of *conservation.*"*

This is what NFA is striving for, conservation of our natural resources by eliminating the exploitative features of our agriculture. We are trying to prevent what we see as a trend toward scientific suicide in this country. Chemical farming methods are exploitative in the extreme. It is mining the soil with synthetic fertilizers and chlorinated hydrocarbon and phosphorus insecticides. We also believe the sale and consumption of overprocessed, devitalized, and chemicalized foods to be just as exploitative as chemical farming. This is but just another facet of the whole picture. Hydrogenated fats, white sugar, white flour, and refined salt are all part of the exploitative economy. If we are to conserve our national health, we will have to begin with personal health.

The U.S. Department of Health, Education, and Welfare has published a bulletin, "Food Facts vs. Food Fallacies," in which they call every belief I have espoused in this book a myth. The U.S. Public Health Department has launched an all-out propaganda campaign to mislead the American people about the state of our national nutrition. They are being supported by the food processors and the chemical trust that makes the poisonous food additives. Science editors, food editors, and medical editors in the daily newspapers have joined their ranks.

They are calling those of us who think otherwise food faddists and quacks. Let's take a close look at this charge. My dictionary defines a fad as "a custom, amusement, or the like, followed for a time with exaggerated zeal; a craze." What, then, is a food faddist? Would you say a faddist is a man who insists on eating bread made from wheat grown on fertile soil and free of toxic pesticides? Or one who demands that the whole grain, containing the vital natural vitamins and minerals, be used in making this bread? For centuries people ate natural foods, and the incidence of metabolic disease was minimal. Was this a passing fad? Or could it be that the milling industry is guilty of quackery and faddism when it removes the vital nutrients before the grain is made into flour? And what of the ones who use poison bleach and add other harmful chemicals to insure keeping quality?

Is it quackery and faddism to be protective of the human

---

*W. C. Lowdermilk, *Conquest of the Land Through 7,000 Years* (U.S. Department of Agriculture Information Bulletin No. 99).

being, and the human race? To be extremely cautious of changes in the food supply that are made strictly for economic gain?

Let's take a look at the source of these cries of quackery and faddism. Modern technology in relatively recent years has brought us the roller mill. The scientist—in this case we should call him a technologist, or hireling scientist—learned how to remove the vitamins and minerals from our cereals. Modern advertising and rapid communication arrived, and—presto!—a new fad was born. Chemists learned how to make synthetic, lifeless vitamins. Presto! another fad. Enriched white bread was next, with its twelve wonderful ways to improve health hawked into the ears of mothers and their children by the new food quacks. "Eat our wonderful breakfast cereal which contains a prize in every box and a cut-out of your favorite Western movie star on the box!" This wondrous news filled both radio and, later, television. Institutes and foundations were formed by the food processors. Millions of dollars poured into their treasuries to create the biggest food fad and promote the most gigantic piece of quackery the world has ever known. It is not difficult to see that they are guilty of "exaggerated zeal" in their efforts to promote their food faddism. Exaggerated zeal. Remember that definition of a fad?

Fortunately, every fad runs its course. We can be optimistic and hope that the dangerous drift toward scientific suicide in this country is also running its course . . . before it is too late.

XIV.

Geministic Bifurcation

By now you know I am not going to slip you a curve in the way of a jawbreaking technical term that goes unexplained. Geministic bifurcation? It sounds like the granddaddy of jawbreakers. Actually it's rather simple. Gemini means twinning or doubling. Bifurcation means cutting in half. Although this sounds like a contradiction in terms, it is not. The concept of geministic bifurcation holds the key to our survival in a polluted, severely overpopulated world, I am convinced. Simply, it is this: *If we would cut waste in half, we could double what we have.*

The concept of geministic bifurcation is not mine, but that of Mendeth E. Smith, director of special projects for International Minerals and Chemical Corporation. Smith poses the crucial question, Can man control his society? Theoretically, if the population doubles by the year 2000 or before, practically everything else will have to double too, if we are to maintain our present standard of living. This means twice as many houses, automobiles, washing machines, baby shoes, and practically everything, including water and food. Most significant of all, we will need twice as much land for highways, airports, home sites, and factory sites. We will need more land for the growing of food. But while the economy possibly could make more of the material objects I have named, nobody can make more land. As a matter of fact, we continue to lose our precious topsoil at an alarming rate, as it annually washes down our rivers into the sea. Facing this dilemma, Smith asks two questions. Can we double those things that need to be doubled? Can we halve those things that need to be halved?

It is easy to see how confusing might be some of the answers to these questions, for they are very difficult ones, perhaps the hardest *Homo sapiens* has had to face. Let us look first at some of the thinking on this subject before we turn to our own workable solution for feeding the starving population of the future.

Many answers to the problem of starvation that faces the future citizens of this world have been proposed. A deficiency of protein is thought by many biochemists to be the chief problem today. This is especially true in some of the so-called underdeveloped nations. The enrichment of cereal grains with synthetic lysine, one of the essential amino acids, has been proposed by Dr. Fredrick J. Stare, chairman of the department of nutrition at Harvard University. Others have similar answers. Paul Deutschman, writing in the International Business Machine Corporation publication,* gives us a quick answer to hunger by informing us that General Electric Company claims to be able to synthesize any of the amino acids. An instant solution to the protein shortage —and a profitable one! To me this is a danger, rather than a solution. The enrichment of the cereal foods of America with synthetic vitamins has already proved to be a failure. Why should enrichment with synthetic proteins be expected to solve any problem?

Although Deutschman seems to believe that the food-and-population crisis has long range solutions, he sees only one quick answer, and that is fertilizer. Chemical fertilizer, of course, and immense quantities of it. He speaks of a "fertilizer revolution": a spontaneous, emergency effort undertaken by various governments, international organizations, private industry, and foundations, to provide a massive increase in the production and use of chemical fertilizer, and thus, to keep half or more of the world from famine. As proof, he offers the old view that fertilizer in large amounts will give a 300 per cent increase in yield. The choice, according to him, is either fertilizer or famine. In support of his idea he summons the words of Dr. Raymond Ewele, vice president for research at New York State University, whom he calls one of the world's leading chemical economists, "that if Asia, Africa, and Latin America are not using quantities of fertilizer

---

*_Think_, November-December, 1966.

approaching 30 million tons by 1980, they are almost certain to be engulfed in widespread famine."

This, to me, is an old, unfeasible idea that fails to answer our growing problems that today demand more imaginative thinking, if we are to solve them. Isn't the fertilizer solution for those three continents just another version of the old story that one dollar spent for fertilizer will return the farmer three dollars? The best thing our government could do to help those farmers in Asia, Africa, and Latin America would be to send some of those Iowa organic farmers to explain to them what commercial fertilizer will eventually do to their land—and to themselves. Synthetic fertilizer rapes and murders the fertility of the soil, and in the end this quick answer will compound the problem of the global population explosion. The end result of chemical farming is always disease, first in the soil and then in the plant and finally in the people who eat this inferior food. The massive use of commercial fertilizer in the so-called underdeveloped nations of the world will bring them the same massive increase in metabolic disease that we already have in America. Massive use of synthetic nitrogen will demand massive use of DDT and other dangerous insecticides, and this will require massive amounts of drugs to alleviate the symptoms of metabolic diseases that are sure to follow. The underdeveloped countries might well be better off if they had never heard of our modern technology. Synthetic fertilizer has not solved the problem in America; it has caused a problem. Thus, it cannot solve the worldwide problem. Because of chemical farming methods, the poisoning of our environment, and the overprocessing of our foods, the American disease and death rate surpasses that in many so-called underdeveloped nations.

We do not claim that malnutrition is the only cause of disease. Proper exercise is certainly essential. Our modern way of hurried stressful city living is a factor in metabolic diseases. Smoking is certainly related to lung cancer, emphysema, and heart disease. Excessive sunburn is dangerous. These are all contributing factors. But our food crisis is at the top of the list.

Another proposed answer to the problem of famine in an exploding population is hydroponics. Hydroponics means dustless farming, a word formed from two Greek roots, *hydro* or water and *ponic* or growth. Instead of good fertile soil as we know it, with micro-organisms in it, this type of agriculture would use gravel, sand, or other dead, inert materials in fiber glass growing beds.

Plants are fed synthetic fertilizers and inorganic nutrients in an electronically-controlled environment that can ignore such variables as soil temperature and rainfall. Artificial light, cooling, and heating are employed. An official of Pan American Hydroponics, Inc., has explained, "The day may come when soil is out of style for growing the foodstuffs that sustain civilization." Well, one can grow beautiful tomatoes and other vegetables by this method, but unfortunately they will not sustain life. Hydroponics is merely carrying the principle of synthetic fertilizer to its dismal, lifeless ultimate conclusion.

A few years ago the new birth control pills were being touted as the answer to the population explosion. Millions of young women all over America and throughout the world have taken the Pill to control the size of their families. At last, it seemed to many, the easy, quick answer! But they spoke too soon. Unfortunately, the mighty Pill had side effects that were not pleasant. A large percentage of American women has discontinued use of the Pill because of these unpleasant side effects. The long range dangers of the Pill are still under intensive investigation. I have never prescribed the modern birth control pill to any of my patients because I have not yet become convinced of its safety. Needless to say, many other physicians doubt the safety of the Pill, also. Its long range effect on the entire endocrine system is still unknown. We do know that the Pill should not be taken indefinitely, and it positively should not be used except under the constant surveillance of a physician. This alone precludes its use in the so-called underdeveloped countries. Therefore, the Pill is not the answer to our worldwide population explosion any more than are the war, pestilence, and disease that eighteenth century economist Malthus foresaw as the only controllers of overpopulation. I predict that the present birth control pill will become but a memory in my own lifetime.

Not only has science failed to curb the exploding population, thus far no good solution has been found to the increasingly critical problem of feeding the growing population. The Malthusian theory is now a fact, rather than theory; war, pestilence, and famine remain the great controllers of population. And in the United States, traffic accidents kill more persons than war does. Modern science with all its technological advances has failed to solve our major problem; in fact, our technological advances in agriculture have actually made the matter worse. The widespread use of agricultural chemicals and commercial fertilizer has fouled the nest of the whole world. Not only the birds, our wildlife, and fresh water fish, but the ocean itself is now contaminated with insecticides and herbicides. Worst of all, our people have become poisoned. The pestilence of cancer, degenerative disease, and even birth defects has already become the scourge of the "enlightened" developed nations of the world.

It is not necessary to merely take my word for this. Dr. Barry Commoner, chairman of the department of botany at Washington University, tells us that the massive opportunities given to modern science and technology include opportunities to make massive mistakes—which we have already witnessed. He has said that "continued pollution of the earth, if unchecked, will eventually destroy the fitness of this planet as a place for human life." The failure of our modern science of agricultural technology and food technology is responsible for many of our troubles. Our people have been taught to have a blind faith in these sciences. A stealthy commercialism has captured many of our scientists, to the detriment of the consumer, and our modern science in agriculture and food technology has not only failed, it has brought us to the brink of destruction.

Is there any hope for the future of our food supply? Is it too late? Is there any answer to our dilemma?

The only workable answer is, I believe, in geministic bifurcation. I don't believe we will ever double our food supply until we learn how to halve our wasteful ways. The first step in solving our problem is to stop waste. We must halt soil erosion both by wind and water. We already know how to prevent erosion, but billions instead of millions should be appropriated by the Congress to put proven conservation practices to work on the land. Small watershed protection programs are proceeding at a snail's pace. We must not only learn to use every available acre according to its capability, we must also put these practices into effect. Covering suitable acres with trees and grasses and restoring the fertility of our crop lands with organic matter will be necessary to solve this problem of erosion.

And we must *stop wasting waste!* All animal manures, garbage, even sewage sludge can be, and must be, composted and returned to the land. If we could halve the waste of these materials, we could double the fertility of our soils and thus double the food supply. We condemn the people of India for burning their cattle dung and using it for fuel; yet how can we justifiably condemn them when we waste so much of it here in America? Hundreds of feedlots have the problem of disposal of the mountains of manure that accumulate. Recently a farmer told me that he could get manure spread on his farm for only $3 per ton. But the county agent told him that it was not worth it and that, furthermore, it would cause weeds and undesirable grasses to grow on his pasture. Our farmers have been told by the experts at the agricultural colleges that commercial fertilizer is much cleaner, cheaper, and easier to use than these *waste* products. As a result, chicken litter and cattle manure are wasted and present problems when they ought to be the key to the solution. The garbage that piles up in our great urban centers is also wasted. It represents the life of our soils out on the farms. Great cities spend fortunes to burn or bury it. We are wasting waste with a vengeance, and it must stop if America is to feed even itself. All this material must be composted and returned to the soil. We must double the fertility of our soils, and the addition of properly composted organic matter is the chief way in which to accomplish this life-saving measure.

There is hope. The idea of composting city garbage, which has already proved to be economical in Europe, is beginning to catch on in America. But we must also stop the wasteful practice of treating our raw rock phosphate and potash with acids before applying them to the land. The proper use of limestone, raw rock phosphate, and potash, with their trace minerals, will be necessary on some lands.

There is another wasteful practice that America must change. We must learn to stop wasting the precious vitamins and minerals that occurs when we overprocess and devitalize our food. We must learn to stop the degermination of our cereals. The whole world needs to learn this lesson. The *quality* of our foods could be doubled if we halved this wasteful practice. With modern refrigeration and transportation it could be done. The Swiss with their Migros movement have already proved that it can be done. Imagine what a groceryman with vision could do in this country!

We need to halve—or bring to the vanishing point!—the poisoning of our foods, in order to double their safety. We need to cut in half or more the use of synthetic nitrogen, DDT, and other dangerous cancer-causing insecticides and weedicides. This is one area where cutting in half isn't enough; we must cut these out entirely. They have fouled our nest and threaten our very existence on this planet. It is necessarily going to be a gradual process, but we must begin as dramatically as we can.

In general, this solution is a simple one, but I hope one will not be misled by its seeming simplicity. Barbara E. Wright, an associate biochemist at the Huntington Laboratories of Harvard University, has said that "the correct hypothesis for the solution of a problem often turns out to be the least complicated one that can be thought of at the time." Experience has taught us that nature operates in the shortest way possible.

The only inexhaustible source of wealth is a fertile soil. In the coming age of famine, proper nutrition from a fertile soil will be the first source of wealth. One may be a millionaire or a president and be struck down with a coronary or a cancer and become a poor man, quickly forgotten. But if in the coming years a man can look forward to proper nutrition from a fertile soil, he can expect to enjoy a health that is a wealth of immeasurable quality. If a man physically contributes to the production of that proper nutrition, by working his own farm or even with a backyard garden, he will be all the more fortunate. Meaningful work has long been recognized as essential to man's well-being. It will continue to be necessary in the future, no matter how many push-button gimmicks may be invented.

The backyard garden is coming back to the Soviet Union. It must become popular in America. It must become a way of life all over America—and all over the world. Each of us must do what he can to feed the exploding population. The first step is to begin at home, to help feed oneself and his family. This will be a highly significant step toward doubling the food supply, while halving our waste.

Geministic bifurcation? Let's just call it a long synonym for *survival.*

XV.

It Is Never Too Late

As a regular annual delegate to national conventions of the Soil and Water Conservation District Supervisors, I have in a relatively short time seen the pattern change in regard to chemical farming. In the early 1960s I heard important officials of the U.S. Department of Agriculture extol the virtues of agricultural research as the best tool to help the farmer solve his problems. Increasing yields consistently dominated as a theme of the committee on research that I attended each year. But in the late 1960s pollution problems began to gain the limelight. One year we were told that modern farm chemicals could be dangerous unless they were used according to directions; we were assured, however, they were safe if so used and that they were necessary if we were going to feed an exploding population. This, in itself, represented a slight change in trend.

Then, one year in the late 1960s, the committee on research featured a talk about pollution from industrial wastes and sewage disposal. There was very little about pollution from agricultural chemicals. At the close of the program, the chairman asked if there were any questions.

I had managed to get a front seat. I quickly faced the audience and read from a medical journal this headline: "Nitrogen Fertilizers Held Peril to Infants."

Then I told them what I had read.

"The farmers of America, *through ignorance,* are poisoning little babies!"

It almost broke up the convention. You could have heard a pin drop.

Then I asked the committee, *"When is this mass poisoning going to stop?"*

The chairman quickly regained his composure and called a Dr. Warleigh, chief of the USDA research division, to the platform.

Dr. Warleigh looked me straight in the eye and said, "Dr. Nichols, we are aware of the problem, and we are working on it."

Is it too late to save this nation and our babies from the mass poisoning caused by excessive nitrogen fertilization? Is it too late to save the ecology—and us—from the dangerous pesticides? Is it too late to save us from the fragmenting results of overprocessed foods? Is it too late to control our raging epidemics of cancer, heart disease, and other metabolic disorders?

I think there is yet time. I hope so. More and more, responsible scientists are spreading the bad news about our poisoned world. Each day another discovery documents the NFA story. As the people become aware of the environmental and health crisis that is upon us, I am hopeful that they will react, as individuals and as groups, to curtail this critical poisoning of our food and atmosphere, and to turn back the tide and to help construct a world more in tune with nature than the world we have been building for generations to ravage nature.

Scientists are concerned with the survival of our species. We have men like Dr. LaMont C. Cole, professor of ecology at Cornell University, and Dr. Barry Commoner, at Washington University at St. Louis, who are leaders in the scientific world in heralding the facts of this imperiled world. Dr. Cole, reading a paper at an annual meeting of the American Association for the Advancement of Science, propounded the question, Can the World Be Saved? He answered it with a scant affirmative, depending almost entirely on the ability of "natural scientists, social scientists, and political leaders . . . to communicate with each other and with the general public." Dr. Cole has hit upon the crux of the matter. Without this vital communication, the country is likely to continue to wallow in confusion.

At the same annual meeting, held in New York, Dr. Commoner read a paper, "Informing the Public: The Duty of the

Scientist in the Environmental Crisis," in which he said: "The environment, which as an integrated whole supports human life, is being stressed to the point of collapse. I believe that we are approaching, in our time on this planet, a crisis which may destroy its suitability as a place for human society. But I believe that we have also learned that the environmental crisis *can* be resolved if we in the scientific community fulfill our duty to inform our fellow citizens about it."

Dr. Commoner has been doing his share of work in this vital role of informing the public. In that same speech he warned that "widespread use of nitrates to fertilize soils may be affecting human health—baby foods especially may be affected." Dr. Commoner's warning was timely. In the last twenty-five years there has been a twelve-fold increase in the use of synthetic nitrogen. The increased concentration of nitrate in food grown on soils so heavily fertilized *is* dangerous to human health. In a study at the University of Missouri Agricultural Experiment Station, investigators found beets and spinach contaminated with as much as 0.8 per cent nitrate nitrogen. An infant, if fed a two-ounce jar of this contaminated baby food, would get 40 milligrams of nitrate. Public health officials have stated that nitrate nitrogen in excess of 12 milligrams daily is in excess. In the presence of certain intestinal bacteria, nitrate is converted to nitrite, which is even more toxic to the infant. Nitrite combines with hemoglobin to form methemaglobin, which cannot adequately transport oxygen to the tissues of the infant. Methemoglobinemia results. This is the blue baby syndrome. We have discussed it earlier in the case of the "hot wells" in Iowa. Unless promptly and adequately treated, the afflicted infant dies.

I think that nitrate poisoning could be a factor in the baffling new disease described as "crib deaths." Babies, who apparently are perfectly well and happy, are put to bed and then are found dead in bed the next morning. Autopsies have failed to determine the cause of death. This is the Number One cause of death in babies under the age of two years. One of 350 babies dies a crib death. Some say cause of death is unknown; others suspect a virus. Some physicians believe crib deaths are caused by infections of the larynx, trachea, and bronchial tubes; *laryngotracheo bronchitis* is the medical term. Some advise that babies be kept away from drafts, be kept warm, and be kept out of contact with persons with colds or influenza. But many of the babies have no indications of upper respiratory infection! Therefore, the role of synthetic nitrates from fertilizer seems more suspect to me and I advise the parents of small children accordingly. I tell mothers to refrain from buying commercial baby foods, but to buy a blender and feed the baby natural, poison-free food grown on fertile soil. It has been my experience that babies fed this way will refuse to eat poison commercial baby foods.

The threat to babies becomes more grave each year. A few years ago the tolerance level of DDT for milk was set at zero by our public health officials. This was supposed to protect our infants, most of whom no longer have the privilege of nursing their mothers' breasts. But now since most of the dairy feed contains DDT it has been almost impossible to find milk that does not contain DDT. This posed a tremendous problem for the Food and Drug Administration (FDA) and the U.S. Department of Agriculture. It was against their regulations to sell milk that contained DDT; yet most of the milk being sold contained the poison. The FDA, under pressure from agricultural interests, eventually changed the regulation and established a legal tolerance for DDT in milk. Thus, it became legal for babies to drink poison milk. Is there any escape for babies, regardless of where they get their milk? Even human mother's milk now contains DDT, as a result of the DDT residues in the human diet.

Obviously, it seems to me, the manufacture of DDT should be prohibited. Setting a "safe" tolerance by the FDA is not enough. The FDA does not have enough inspectors to insure the safety of our foods. In a recent year, 680,000 pounds of butter was confiscated in Arizona because it contained too much DDT. I shudder to think of the millions of pounds of poison butter that is being consumed now because there has been no adequate inspection.

Inevitably the economic questions arise when a discussion of this sort is under way. Without a doubt, the profits of the agricultural chemical industry would be threatened if we curtailed or halted the manufacture and sale of the highly-dangerous poisons and chemicals. But which is more important? Must one man get rich because another gets sick—or dies? We need to get this whole controversy into proper focus. The health of this nation, and our people, should rank *first.*

One European country after another has banned DDT and other dangerous pesticides. Wisconsin and Arizona have banned it. The Department of the Interior has eliminated its use on public lands. The U.S. government has fluctuated between banning it and banning the ban. DDT is a cancer-causing chemical. It must be banned in every state in America. Alden, Dieldrin, Endrin, Heptachlor, and Chlordane should also be banned everywhere. It is not enough to warn the American housewife that the pesticide strip should not be used in the kitchen. There is *no* safe way to use them. Use according to directions? There can be no safe directions for them, if we are concerned with our children's health, and our own. All of us already have too much DDT stored in our bodies, and there is scientific evidence that increased storage of these persistent compounds may be found in persons suffering from chronic disorders such as portal cirrhosis, carcinoma, and hypertension. Studies conducted in France suggest that these insecticides even pass the placental barrier that normally protects the foetus from poisons. Thus, our babies are being born with DDT poisoning! Mother's milk contains DDT, and most of the cow's milk used to feed the majority of our infants has DDT in it. That is why this deadly, cancer-causing poison, and others like it, must be banned. There is no other way to protect our babies. Furthermore, these chemicals are vitamin antagonists and enzyme inhibitors, and they are related directly to malnutrition.

The evidence is becoming clearer and clearer every day now. We are faced with the rapid loss of what is perhaps our most precious freedom, the freedom to be healthy. What is a man who is not healthy? How can a baby enjoy life, enjoy his childhood, if he is not healthy? A baby born today in America does not have the freedom to breathe poison-free air, to drink poison-free water, or to eat poison-free food. Unless we have the freedom to enjoy health, and the freedom to eat natural, poison-free food in an unpolluted atmosphere, we will enjoy our other freedoms less. A friend of mine has told me, "I'd rather be sick in America than healthy behind the Iron Curtain." Perhaps he has a point, but as long as we're choosing, I would prefer to be healthy in America.

I'm satisfied it isn't too late to do something about this critical state of our national health. I have seen dramatic changes in my own patients' health, and I believe the same thing could happen on the national level if we would but reduce the toxicity and the fragmentation of our environment and food supply.

I've seen it happen time after time in dealing with patients. One of the best examples I know is a golf professional from Dallas. He called me from Dallas a few years ago; his fingers had become so stiff he couldn't get them around a golf club. He had heard that I might be able to help him.

For a pro golfer, his health problem was quite a serious one. He had a form of arthritis that had caused stiffness in his fingers so that he was no longer able to grip a golf club. He had been to several doctors, had had a complete physical examination with the usual tests and X-rays, and had taken the usual remedies. But he still couldn't use a golf club as once he had. For a man with a wife and three children who was accustomed to a good standard of living, this health problem was more than a painful inconvenience; it was a threat to his whole way of life and well-being and to his ability to produce income.

He made a ten a.m. appointment at the clinic. I marked off the appointment book for the rest of the morning, to give him my full attention. He and his wife drove in from Dallas, slightly under 200 miles, and I wanted them to get their money's worth.

I recognized when they came into my office that day that they were both skeptical. For that, I couldn't blame them. After all, they had never been in my clinic or seen me before that day. But I cancelled all my appointments and spent the whole day with him. I went over in very careful detail the whole story of proper nutrition. I drew a picture of the grain of wheat and told him how to eat. Then I prescribed 50 milligrams of vitamin B_6 for his stiff fingers.* Vitamin B_6 is known to be essential in more than thirty different biochemical reactions at the cellular level. He was eating the ordinary country club diet, snacking a great deal; so he was very deficient in the water-soluble B vitamins. Vitamin B_6 is water soluble and thermolabile, or subject to damage by heat. Then I took him and his wife to my farm, where I put some fresh, organic, unsprayed vegetables into his car. I also took them to our NFA national headquarters near Atlanta. I spent two hours showing and telling them the whole NFA story that afternoon. I gave them what I call the VIP Tour.

Three weeks later, he was back on the golf course. He could grip a golf club and by then he was on proper nutrition and the stiffness in his hands had subsided.

But as they left that afternoon, even though I had spent

---

*A classic book on this whole subject is *The Doctor Who Looked at Hands* (Vantage Press, New York) by my friend, Dr. John M. Ellis of Mt. Pleasant, Texas.

hours with that patient, I still felt I had not completely convinced his wife. This is most important, in medicine as in other fields. This was particularly important in his case, for, after all, one's wife usually has quite a lot to say about one's diet. I could just tell, without words to tip me off, that I had not sold his wife on the idea of natural food. After a while I've developed a sort of special sense about those things.

Several months later when I was in a Dallas department store, a woman walked up to me and tapped me on the shoulder. It was the wife. She proceeded to tell me how well he was doing. He was healthy and a completely changed man in every way.

"He's a better man and a good husband," she said. "He used to feel bad. He was grouchy. Now he's pleasant and a good father and husband."

"You know," I said, "when you left my office that day, I somehow felt you were still not completely convinced."

She laughed and said, "How did you know? The first thing I said to Bill when we got in the car was, 'I don't see how anything that simple can do that much good!' You're right; I was skeptical, but I am no longer."

But something that simple did do that much good. It's typical of the NFA story. It's a simple story, really. It further points up my contention that nationally, and even internationally, it is never too late. What it did for Bill, it can do for millions like him.

There is a sequel to Bill's story. That winter, he was on the program committee of the Texas Professional Golf Association (PGA), and he asked me to make the same speech to its convention that I had made to him. The speech was scheduled for a Monday morning in January in Waco, Texas.

My wife, Mildred, and I drove to Waco in a snow and sleet storm the preceding Sunday afternoon. In spite of the inclement weather, 150 golfers attended. The program started at nine a.m., with each speaker allotted an hour. I was the third speaker, scheduled for eleven a.m. The first speaker droned to a dry conclusion at 10:45 a.m. The audience was getting fidgety, and I will never forget how nervous I was. There was only one hour and fifteen minutes until lunch—and another one-hour speech would precede mine! How could I sum up my Concept of Totality in the fifteen minutes he would leave me? The only consolation I had was that I had already made arrangements to introduce myself, which would enable me to utilize every second of the time I did expect to have.

I needn't have worried, as it turned out. As the first speaker sat down, the master of ceremonies stood up and announced that the second speaker hadn't arrived. Whatever had delayed him, whether he was snowbound or not, I was not exactly unhappy over it. As a result, I had one hour and ten minutes for my own speech.

My audience was composed of young golfers. It was getting near lunchtime. The first speech had caused their interest to wander. I sensed I was about to lose my audience. They were restive, and my speech topic as listed in the program, "A Concept of Totality," had not proved inspiring enough to make them sit upright and cheer when I strode to the podium.

Since it was already understood I would introduce myself, I forthwith identified myself and said, "The program says 'A Concept of Totality' is my subject, but instead I'm going to speak on 'How to Live to Be 100, Get Shot by a Jealous Husband, and Still Go to Heaven.'

"I'm also going to tell you how to get the stiffness out of your fingers and how to get your fingers around a golf club and lower your score."

With that promise, they all sat up with piqued interest, and I had an audience for the next hour and ten minutes. I told them in condensed form what I had told Bill several months earlier. In effect, I delivered my original "Concept of Totality" speech, and they listened to it carefully because I was talking about their bread and butter.

The truth is that millions of other Americans are much more afflicted than any of these athletes and don't realize that they are victims of a national biological blight that has stricken America. The late Dr. Tom Douglas Spies summed up the changed situation in health care when he wrote: "Today germs are not our principal enemy. Our chief medical adversary is what I consider a disturbance of the inner balance of the constituents of our tissues, which are built from and maintained by necessary chemicals in the air we breathe, the water we drink, and the food we eat. Persons who are afflicted with 'rheumatism' or 'cancer,' for example, are not the victims of germs but of altered chemistry. For a generation we have worked on the concept that our cells are never static and that in time they must be replaced in varying degrees by the nutrients obtained from food. More specifically, our working hypothesis has been that all disease is chemical and, when we knew enough, chemically correctable." Then he went on to say: "A large part of human disease is chemical rather than bacterial in origin, and in diseases of chemical origin the trouble may be either excess or deficiency—the effect on the patient is a general biological blight, and a spectacular response follows the administration of complex foodstuffs."*

It is, I think, in the field of metabolic disease that quality food can play a highly significant role in both prevention and treatment. Even in the area of acute infection, the importance of proper nutrition is now being recognized. Dr. Seymour Lionel Halpern has written: "The ability of a patient to recover from an illness, injury, or operation is closely related to his previous and current nutrient supply. Rare indeed is the patient who cannot be aided by proper nutritional guidance, since *nutrition is probably the most important environmental factor affecting health and disease.*"** Good nutrition will help to insure rapid wound healing following surgery, burns, or radiation exposure. Proper nutrition is not only important in preventing weight disturbances and specific deficiency disease, it also has an equally vital role in maintaining high grade health. In a non-specific manner, nutrition participates in the prophylaxis against most acute infections and, when used as an adjunct in therapy, shortens the duration of convalescence of virtually all pathologic processes. Halpern maintains that for an optimum effect, there must be a proper balance and proportion among nutrients, and *all* the nutrients utilized by the tissues must be available to the cell *simultaneously* and *in balance*. Does this sound familiar?

Americans have come to believe that they can go down to a clinic and get a checkup with X-rays, get a prescription, and take it down to the drugstore—they believe that they can buy health. But they can't do it. They can buy relief from symptoms sometimes, and might even prolong life, but they'll still be sick. The American people must be made to realize that they can't buy health like this. Health is bought with daily living, not with money, and in order to save every American, and this great coun-

---

*"Some Recent Advances in Nutrition," *Journal of the American Medical Association*, June 7, 1958.

***Annals of the New York Academy of Science*, Oct. 28, 1955.

try, from preventable metabolic disease, this and other changes must be brought about. We must recognize, before it is too late, that chemical farming and overprocessing of foods in a poisoned environment have placed us, individually and as a nation, in a crisis. We must face and overcome this crisis by restoring the soil's fertility through intelligent organic farming methods, as well as by demanding, and getting, the end of fragmentation and chemical additives in food and the elimination of poisons in our daily diet. If this nation can send men to the moon, it should have enough imagination to market profitably enough natural, poison-free foodstuffs to set this country on a more healthful course. Is not our health our greatest national asset? Is it not each person's greatest personal asset?

The preservation of our environment has become the political issue of the 1970s. Democrats and Republicans alike have jumped on the bandwagon. Even third party candidates are for clean air, pure water, and good poison-free food. Newspapers and magazines are filled with stories about pollution and the dire consequences that are sure to follow. Everyone is concerned about pollution, and certainly everyone should be.

But one of the most damaging forms of pollution is our food pollution. The American people can never enjoy proper nutrition until they learn the fundamental value of natural foods of high quality. Snacks made from white flour, white sugar, glucose, and hydrogenated fats must be abandoned. The Five D's—Delicious, Delectable, Death-Dealing Desserts—made from these same dead foods must be abandoned.

I am calling for a revolution. There must be a revolution in the eating habits of America, if we are to save her—and us. America today is starving for a good loaf of whole grain bread, and that's just the beginning. We must eradicate the dangerous chemicals and poisons from our environment and from our food. We must halt the risky fragmentation of our foods. We must eliminate all sources of pollution. We must, in short, initiate programs aimed at producing natural, organically-grown, poison-free food for all America, and every citizen must do his share in bringing this about. He can work with his elected representatives in government, at both the local and higher levels; he can organize local groups; he can join Natural Food Associates, and he can see that he and his family get proper nutrition. If he is a farmer, or if he has enough space for a backyard garden, he can personally institute a system of organic farming. In many areas of the highly complex society we live in, individuals are often lost and may count for little, but in this grave health crisis that we face in America today, there is a great deal that an individual—just one person—can accomplish. To begin with, he can save himself and his family. If he does nothing else, this example of health will not be lost on his neighbors.

I have never been a pessimist. I have often watched the sun set in the west. Many times it was beautiful. Sometimes it was obscured by dark clouds. But, always, I knew that in the morning that great sun would rise again in the east.

In our nation we are seeking our way through a long night of darkness.

When the sun rises—if it does—in the east tomorrow, will it be on a sea of ignorance, or on a mountain of health and hope?

The answer depends on you.

Recommended Books

The following books are recommended, and they can be obtained from the NFA Bookstore, Atlanta, Texas 75551.

Carson, Rachel. *Silent Spring.* (pb) Fawcett Books, Greenwich, Conn.

Cheraskin, E., M.D., D.M.D. and Ringsdorf, W. M., Jr., D.M.D. *New Hope for Incurable Diseases,* Exposition Press Inc., New York.

Cocannouer, Joseph. *Nature and You.* Natural Food Associates, Atlanta, Texas.

Cocannouer, Joseph. *Organic Gardening and Farming.* (pb) Arco Books, New York.

Cocannouer, Joseph. *Water and the Cycle of Life.* The Devin-Adair Company, Old Greenwich, Conn.

Cocannouer, Joseph. *Weeds: Guardians of the Soil.* The Devin-Adair Company, Old Greenwich, Conn.

Davis, Adelle. *Let's Get Well.* Harcourt, Brace & World, New York.

Ellis, John M., M.D. *The Doctor Who Looked at Hands.* (pb) Arco Books, New York.

Graham, Frank, Jr. *Since Silent Spring.* (pb) Fawcett Books, Greenwich, Conn.

Howard, Sir Albert. *The Soil and Health.* (pb) Schocken Books, New York.

Hunter, Beatrice Trum. *Consumer Beware.* Simon and Schuster, New York.

Hunter, Beatrice Trum. *Gardening Without Poisons.* (pb) Berkley, New York.

Longwood, William. *Poisons in Your Food* (pb) Pyramid, New York.

Martin, W. Coda, M.D. *A Matter of Life: Blueprint for a Health Family.* The Devin-Adair Company, Old Greenwich, Conn.

McCarrison, Sir Robert and Sinclair, H. M. *Nutrition and Health.* Faber and Faber, London, England.

Miller, Fred D., D.D.S. *Open Door to Health.* The Devin-Adair Company, Old Greenwich, Conn.

Natural Food and Farming. (monthly magazine) Natural Food Associates, Atlanta, Texas.

NFA Chapter of Albuquerque. *Avant Garde Cookbook.* Natural Food Associates, Atlanta, Texas.

Philbrick, John and Helen. *The Bug Book.* Philbrick, Wilkinsonville, Mass.

Philbrick, Helen and Gregg, Richard. *Companion Plants.* The Devin-Adair Company, Old Greenwich, Conn.

Picton Lionel, M.D. *Nutrition and the Soil.* The Devin-Adair Company, Old Greenwich, Conn.

Price, Weston A., D.D.S., F.A.C.D. *Nutrition and Physical Degeneration.* Price-Pottenger Foundation, Santa Monica, California.

Storer, John H. *The Web of Life.* (pb) Signet Books, New York.

Stout, Ruth. *Gardening Without Work.* The Devin-Adair Company, Old Greenwich, Conn.

Wickenden, Leonard. *Gardening With Nature.* (pb) Fawcett-Books, Greenwich, Conn.

Williams, Roger, Ph.D. *Nutrition Against Disease.* Pitman Publishing Co., New York.

Index